Contents

Setting the Record Straight

I love dance! Once you are a dancer, the feeling and appreciation for it never leaves you. As a former dancer, I know how hard dancers work and what a tremendous gift they have—one that needs to be shaped and nurtured from young years. Remember, the dancer's body is a miraculous instrument—one that needs to be both fed and cared for properly.

When I was a young jazz and modern dancer, no one really knew what proper nutrition was. There were many fads, myths, and wives' tales circulating about the dance world. We really didn't have access to good information about how to stay both lean and strong. As a result, being young and not knowing where to turn, I didn't nourish myself as well as I could have, and it literally stopped my career short at the young age of thirty-six. Had I known what I know today, I probably would have extended my career at least another ten years, not to mention being able to perform even better when I did dance.

The end of dance was not the end of me. I became an ACE-certified group exercise instructor and personal trainer and have been teaching in New York's fitness industry for over twenty-five years and continue to do so. However, I knew I needed more knowledge to be able to work professionally in the field of wellness.

I entered graduate school and earned a master's degree in clinical nutrition from New York University. As a registered dietitian (RD) and nutritionist for the Ailey School and having worked with the New York City Ballet's Wellness team for two years. I have had the honor of teaching young dancers the basics of nutrition for dance and hope to pass this information on to all dancers. Each person is unique and should be assessed properly.

As you probably know, the dance world has changed quite a bit since I was young in terms of advocating proper nutrition, but there are still many misconceptions about food, weight, and what is just plain healthy for you as a dancer. Remember, the only person qualified to discuss nutrition with you is not your aunt, another dancer, a physical therapist, your trainer, your favorite magazine or Hollywood star, but a registered dietitian (RD). Only an RD has the education, experience and background to teach you what is right for you. An RD has a license to practice dietetics and will be your best source of good and reliable information that will keep you healthy and keep you dancing for many years to come. Licensed nutrition professionals are required to possess a minimum of a bachelor's degree and usually a master's degree. Course work is heavily science-based including chemistry, biology, and biochemistry, along with food and nutritional sciences. Once course work and graduation are done, the completion of a hospital internship must take place as well as passing a national licensing exam. Utilizing the right source of nutrition information is critical for you to receive the information you need to make choices right for you without a focus on "being thin" as the end all and be all of everything. So get your information ONCE from the proper source and forget the rest.

My wish for you is that this handbook serves you as a simple but thorough daily guide to educate you on how to eat for your health, for dance, for injury prevention, for endurance, for stamina, and for the long term. As you know, eating right means a healthy and beautifully balanced strong body and long career for you. It will dispel myths and empower you to make decisions that are right for YOU!

Read on, enjoy. And as the great jazz legend and my teacher Luigi used to say to us in class every day, "Never stop moving."

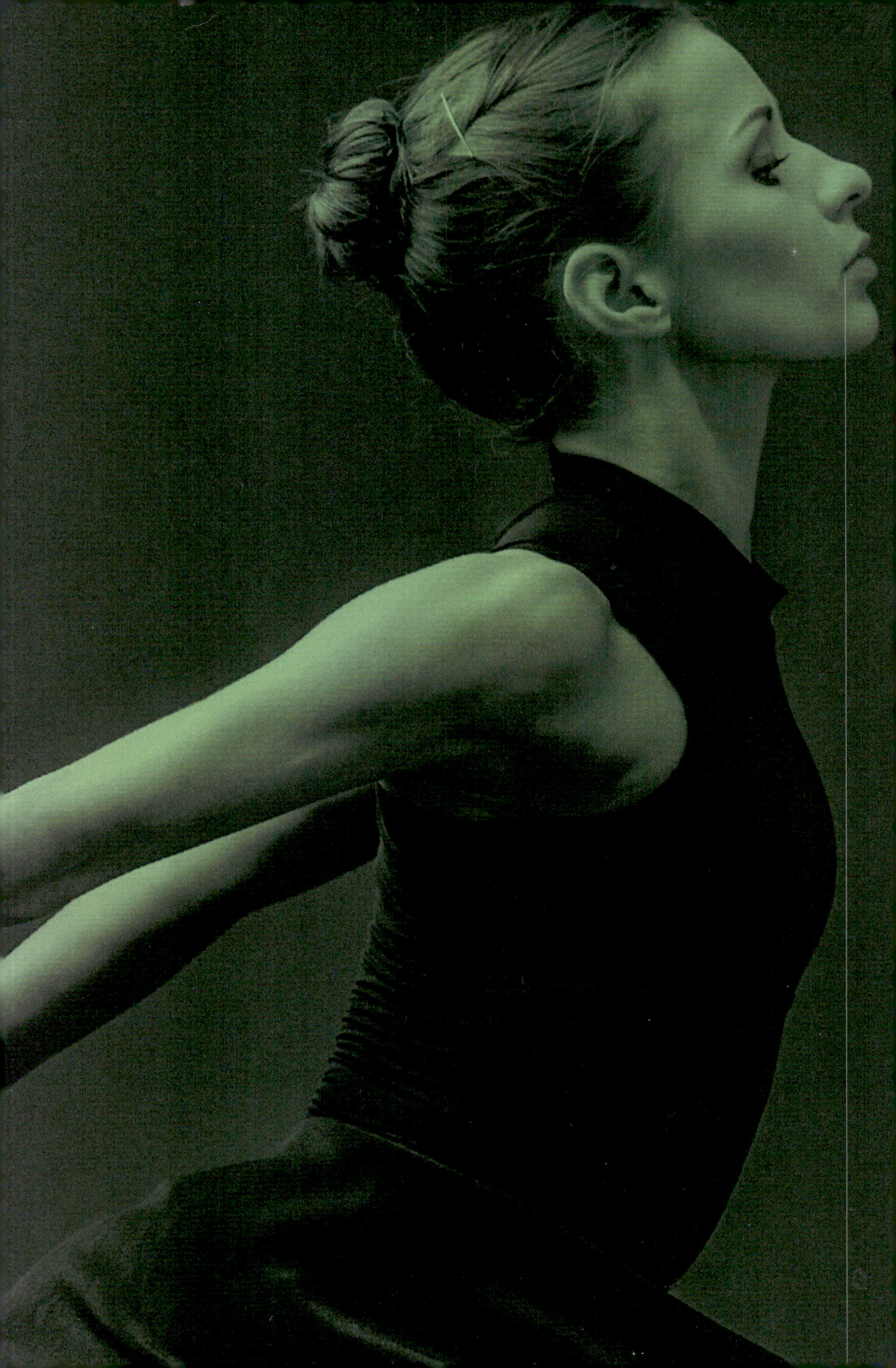

How to Use This Book

This book was written for YOU! It is a guidebook and workbook for today's dancer to determine what is right for you! Use the information as it applies to you and know that if you can follow the guidelines 80% of the time, the rest of the 20% of the time will not affect your health in a negative way. In other words, don't live in a "food prison"! All foods can fit, even your favorites! Do the best you can on most days and forget the rest. No one is perfect, not even registered dietitians!

There are two ways to use this guidebook. You can read it from beginning to end. As each chapter builds on the next, this will probably be the most comprehensive way of accumulating new knowledge. However, you can also read it on a chapter-by-chapter basis not necessarily in order. Each chapter is made to stand on its own. The first four chapters give you background and reference for the others. Do what is right for you. When finished reading, you can keep it on your shelf or in your dance bag as a handy reference in case you forget something.

You can put the recommendations into practice in a general way, or you can go to the next level and make your own personal calculations and/or follow a menu plan. It is totally up to you. Either way will provide you with a better guide to a healthier body.

Take note of the quick tips, fast facts, key notes, and chapter reviews. They will give you easy snapshots of information and will be easy to follow and give you simple ways to absorb and use the suggestions. You don't have to twist yourself into a pretzel to have a healthy diet! Make small changes over time, and you will reap big rewards. The chapter reviews can be printed and given out as handouts for dancers.

I have tried to provide you with practical information and to give you tools to make your dance day easier. There is no sense walking around with a calculator trying to keep track of protein and fat grams. You have more important things to do, like DANCE!

I sincerely hope that this will be the last book you ever need on sports nutrition and nutrition for the dancer. My recommendations are based on industry standards and science, not folk myth or personal hearsay.

There are lots of other links and websites to good information that are professional and useful in addition to sample menu plans and meal and snack suggestions in the appendix. I hope you enjoy this book, and that it helps you have a long, healthy and injury-free career.

And as my jazz teacher and dance legend Luigi always told us in class every day, "Never stop moving!"

Introducing Our Dancers

You may relate to our two dance characters Callie and Gregory. They have the same questions as you do! Learn how they make small changes to their diets and reap big rewards. After all, they want to eat right and dance right!

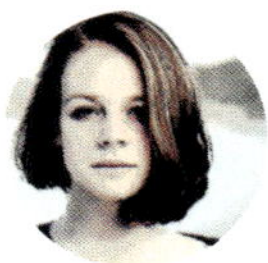

Callie
17 years old

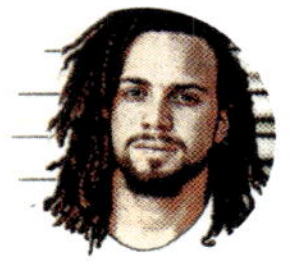

Gregory
20 years old

Callie is a 17 year old female dancer from Georgia, who is doing a summer dance intensive in Chicago. This is her first time away from home and is sharing an apartment with two other girls. She is dancing from 9am to 5pm and is having a difficult time keeping her energy up and just fitting food in during her busy day even though she has a lunch break and some snack breaks. She is feeling tired and needs to sleep more, but she is so excited about the experience she finds it difficult to wind down at night. Also some of the girls in the intensive are talking about supplements for energy and although she is intrigued she is afraid of taking anything and wonders if she should. All in all she hopes this book will answer her questions and help her learn and be healthy. See her progress through each chapter.

Gregory is a 20 year old male dancer from Boston who has moved to New York to audition for Broadway. He is sharing an apartment with 2 other actor/dancers. He is also concerned with having enough energy. He wants to also build muscle to improve his stamina and partnering abilities. He is just learning to cook but also needs help with eating out healthfully as he spends his days auditioning and being out and about. He has heard about "cleansing" and has questions about whether this practice will keep him healthy. He has heard many conflicting ideas about what dancers need to be strong, and is looking forward to separating fact from fiction by reading this book. See how his understanding progresses through each chapter. You may be just like him!

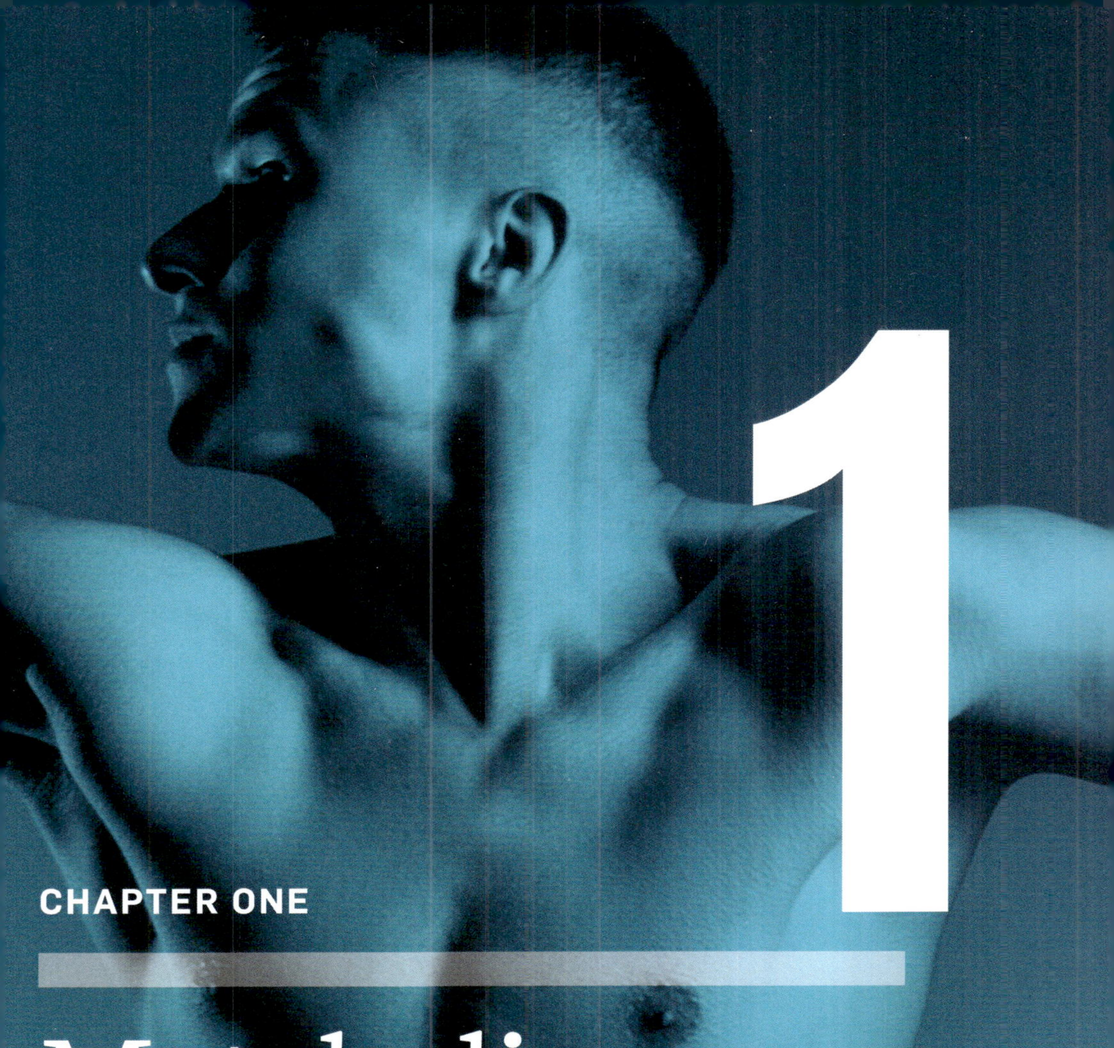

Metabolism and Calories – Mystery No More

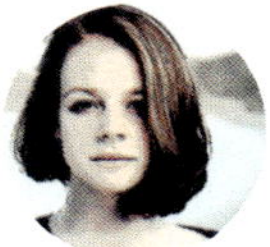

Callie is hearing all kinds of talk at her summer intensive. So many dancers are worried about eating too many calories, and most don't know what is enough for them. She has never counted calories and wonders if she is getting enough to dance well. What should she do? Are you like her? Do you wonder if you have a slow metabolism? Here are some answers that will put your mind at ease:

What in the world is this thing called metabolism? Everyone talks about it, and most dancers (and people in general) think they have a "slow" metabolism. That is absolutely NOT the case with dancers and here is why.

How do I get these needed calories?

They come from all foods and beverages that we eat and drink. Each food and beverage has a different amount of calories. We want to learn to choose the healthiest calories from foods that provide vitamins, minerals, fiber, protein, carbohydrate, and healthy fat, thereby assuring us that our bodies will benefit by this healthy balance.

Our lifestyle determines our metabolism. Our genes, family history, and how much muscle or lean body mass we have also determines how many calories we need on a daily basis to maintain our weight and overall health. Most dancers are extremely lean and have an abundance of muscle. This muscle weight burns calories all day even in rest and sleep. The more muscle you have, the higher your metabolism. As a dancer, you are a calorie-burning machine, so eating enough is critical for many reasons.

How many calories per day do you need as an active dancer/athlete? We base calorie needs on what we call our basal metabolic rate or BMR. This is the number of calories you need just to keep the brain, nervous system and muscles alive. Generally, most female dancers' BMR amounts to approximately 1,300–1,500 calories per day. Generally, most male dancers' BMR amounts to approximately 1,700–2,000 calories per day. That means that if you just stayed in bed, didn't move, and just stared at the ceiling all day, your body would burn the above calories. That doesn't take into account the calories or energy you need to take class, perform, go to work, deal with stress and just live. Most dancers need another 500–700 calories in addition to their BMR to maintain their weight.

Some definitions:

Metabolic Rate: refers to how many calories your body needs (or burns) to just exist. Our calorie needs for existence are referred to as our basal metabolic rate or BMR.

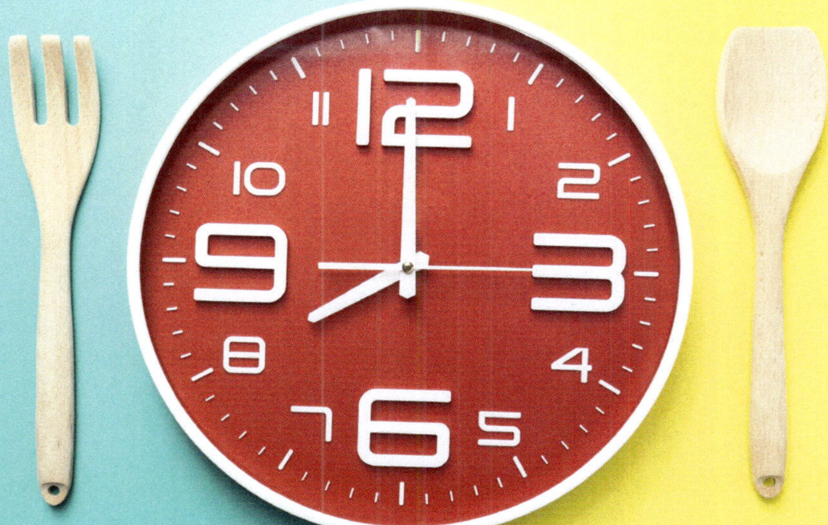

Metabolism: the way in which our body's systems use energy. These systems include digestion, breathing, circulation, muscle building, and brain and nervous system activity.

Calorie: a measure of simply how much energy comes from food. Calories represent not only the fuel you need to dance and live and work but also the fuel you need 24/7 even resting and sleeping. As a dancer, it is important to keep fuel and calories going in for muscular strength and endurance as well as for keeping alert and mentally focused.

That's a lot of food! The dancer's job to maintain good nutrition is to get your eating day started early and be consistent throughout the day. I know this is challenging as your day is filled with classes, work, school, travel, etc., but you will get so much more out of your day by feeding your brain and muscles. Just plan ahead. Use the meal and snack suggestions in the appendix for help in knowing what to pack in your dance bag to be prepared.

Do I need to count calories?

Is it feasible and recommended for dancers to "count" calories? NO! A far more reasonable way to make sure you are getting in enough food in a balanced way is to use the chart I have made for you at different calorie ranges. That way, you just have to know what a "serving" is, and the calories will automatically be correct. Your only job is to read on and learn why you need all the food I am recommending for a dancer's diet, and it will become second nature. Another option would be to just follow a sample menu plan that looks good to you. They are located in the appendix section of this guidebook. Just make it easy for yourself.

Calorie Range
Numbers Represent Approximate Servings of Foods in Food Groups

Calorie Range	Starchy Carbohydrates	Vegetables	Fruits	Dairy	Protein	Fats
1,600 Usually too low for most dancers	5	Unlimited	3	2	7 oz. divided into 2 servings per day	3–4 tsps.
1,800	6	Unlimited	3	3	8 oz. divided into 2 servings per day	4 tsps.
2,100	7	Unlimited	4	3	9 oz. divided into 2 servings per day	5 tsps.
2,400	9	Unlimited	4	3	11 oz. divided into 2 servings per day	5 tsps.
2,700	11	Unlimited	5	3	12 oz. divided into 2 servings per day	5 tsps.
3,000	12	Unlimited	6	4	12 oz. divided into 2 servings per day	6 tsps.

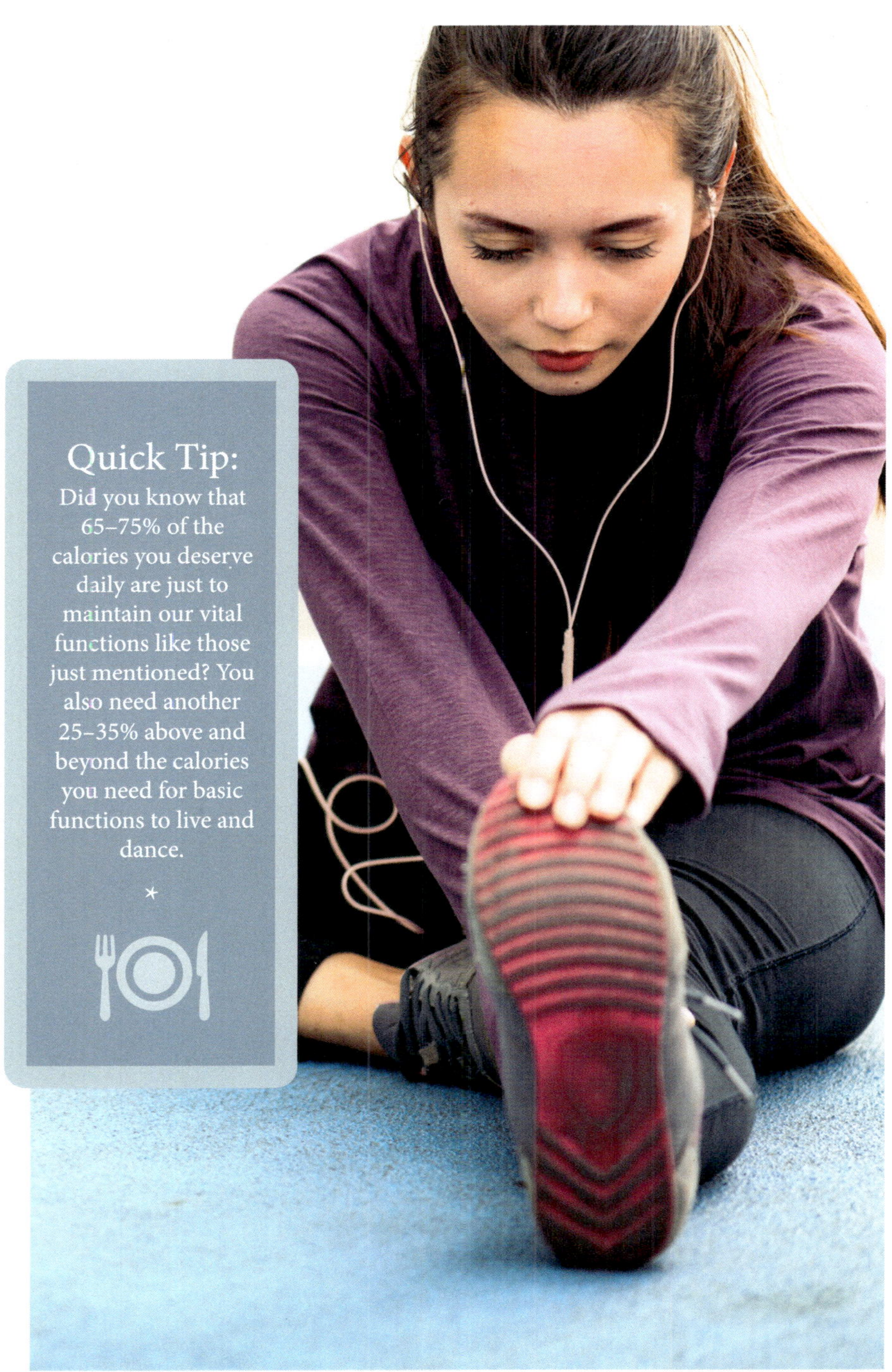

Quick Tip:
Did you know that 65–75% of the calories you deserve daily are just to maintain our vital functions like those just mentioned? You also need another 25–35% above and beyond the calories you need for basic functions to live and dance.

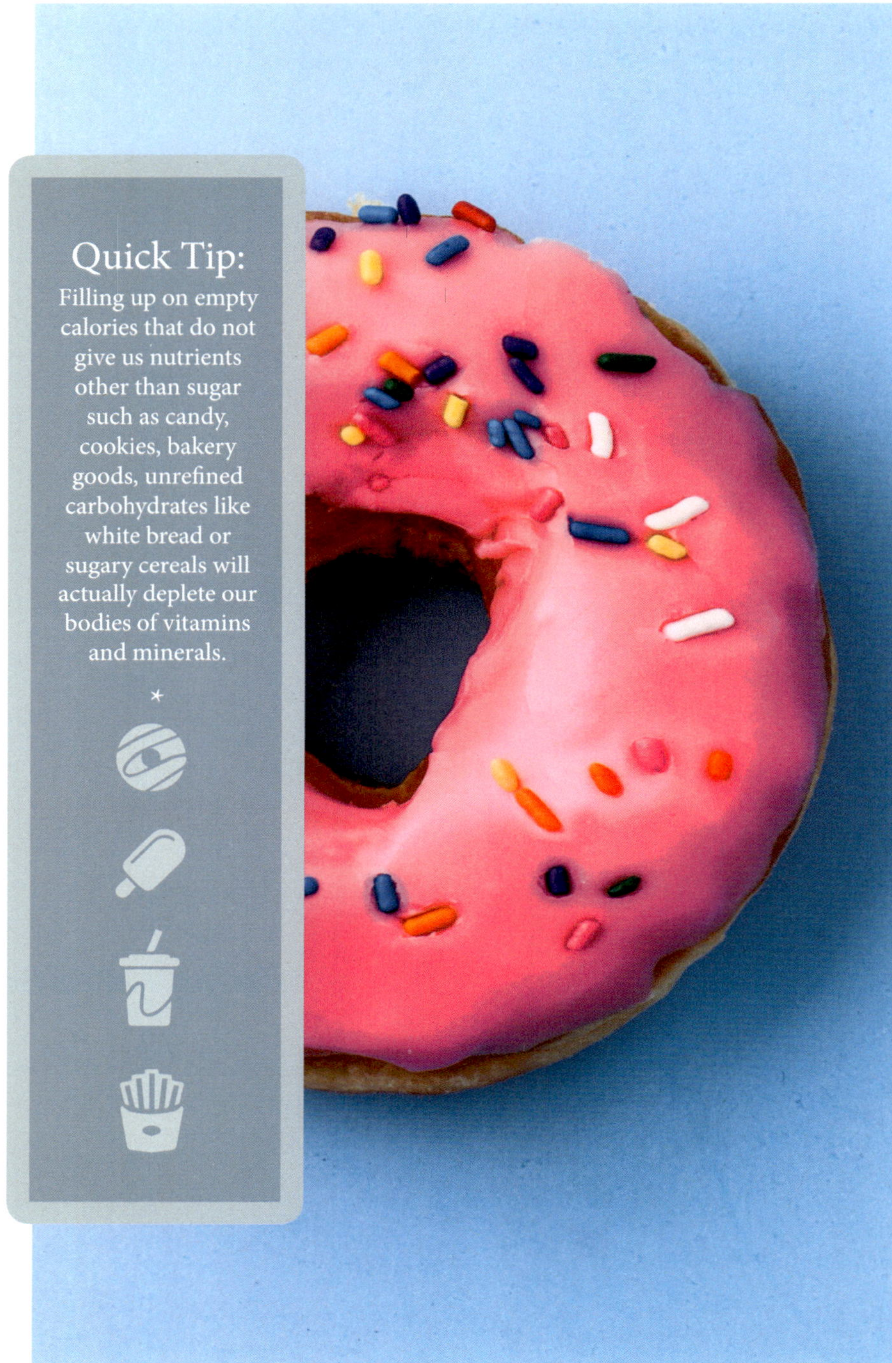
Quick Tip:
Filling up on empty calories that do not give us nutrients other than sugar such as candy, cookies, bakery goods, unrefined carbohydrates like white bread or sugary cereals will actually deplete our bodies of vitamins and minerals.

Here is generally how many calories you need per day:

Female dancers:

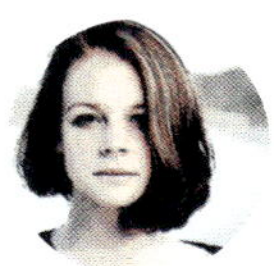

1. Just to maintain their weight, most female dancers age 18 and up would need to consume approximately 1,900–2,300 calories per day.

2. Girls between the ages of 11 and 14 need about 47 calories per kilogram of weight. (Divide your weight in pounds by 2.2 to get weight in kilograms.) That means an 80-pound girl at age 12 or 13 needs about 1,700 calories.

3. Girls between ages 15–18 need about 40 calories per kilogram of weight. That means a 110-pound 18-year-old girl would need at least 2,000 calories per day.

Male dancers:

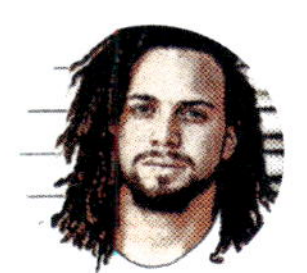

1. Just to maintain their weight, most male dancers age 18 and up need to consume approximately 2,600–2,800 calories or more per day.

2. Boys between the ages of 11 and 14 need about 55 calories per kilogram of weight and those between 15 and 18 need about 45 calories per kilogram of weight. That means that a 140-pound 16-year-old needs close to 2,900 calories. Calorie needs change as growth slows down as you get older; however, dancers are so active that calorie needs almost always stay high.

Fast Facts:

If you do not eat enough calories each and every day, you will lose energy, lose mental focus, crave sugar and be tempted to eat foods that are not good for you.

What is one serving?

Starchy carbohydrates: 80 calories, one ounce dry, 15 grams of carbohydrate
• One slice of bread
• 1 oz. cold cereal
• ½ cup cooked grain, rice, pasta, oatmeal
• 1 small red potato (3 oz.)
• ½ cup peas or corn

Vegetables: 25 calories
• One cup raw salad greens or raw veggies
• ½ cup cooked veggie

Fruits: 60–100 calories
• A small to medium-size fruit
• ½ cup chopped fruit
• 1 cup berries
• ¼ cup dried fruit

Dairy: 80–150 calories
• 1 cup yogurt, milk, soy or almond milks
• 1 oz. cheese
• ¼ cup cottage cheese

Protein: 75–100 calories
• 1 ounce meat, poultry, fish (we usually have 3–4 oz. or more of protein at lunch and dinner)
• Vegetarian equivalents to 1 oz. of meat protein are
1.2 tbsps. nut butter
2.one egg or two egg whites
3.4 oz. tofu
4.½ cup cooked beans or peas

Fats: 1 teaspoon (tsp.) = 45 calories. This refers to the fats used in cooking or as part of salad dressings.

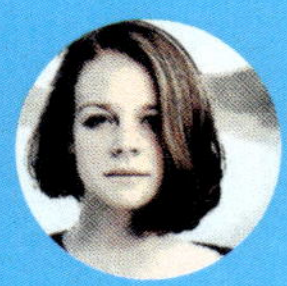

KEY NOTE FROM CALLIE:

Callie asks: What is a healthy balance for me?

Answer: If you visualize your breakfast, lunch or dinner plate, half of it should be covered with vegetables (or perhaps at breakfast fruit can be an option), one quarter of it should be covered with a starchy carbohydrate (like rice or other grain, potato, pasta, bread or crackers), and one quarter of it should be covered with a protein (like lean red meat, poultry, fish, eggs, beans, nuts or soy). Vegetables can be dressed with olive or canola oil for a healthy fat. Fruits and dairy foods (like cheese, milk, or yogurt) can round out a meal or make a snack. See MyPlate guide in appendix.

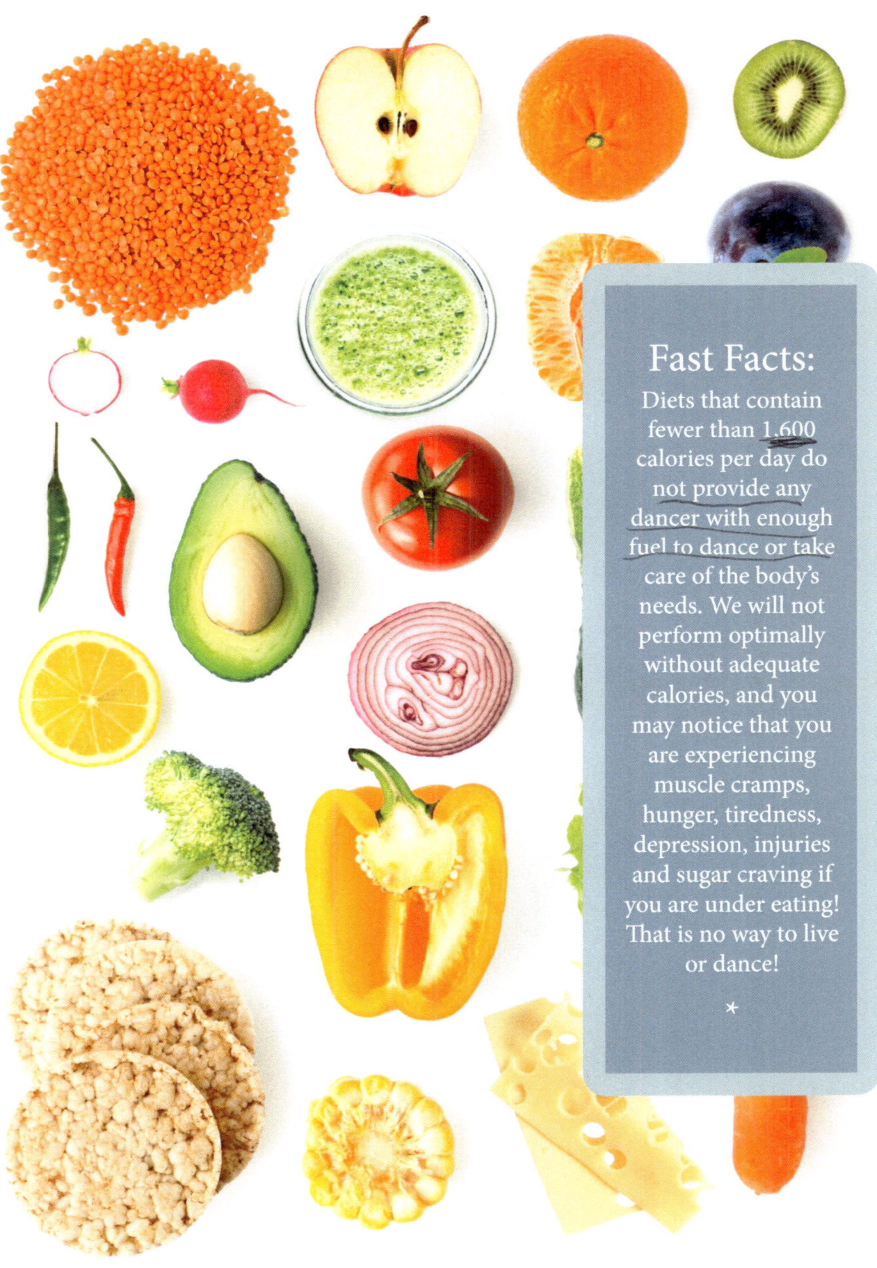

Fast Facts:

Diets that contain fewer than 1,600 calories per day do not provide any dancer with enough fuel to dance or take care of the body's needs. We will not perform optimally without adequate calories, and you may notice that you are experiencing muscle cramps, hunger, tiredness, depression, injuries and sugar craving if you are under eating! That is no way to live or dance!

*

A Model Diet Example:

Say I am Callie, and I want to try to eat around 2,100 calories per day. If I follow the 2,100 calorie chart in terms of servings, here is an example of what I would eat in one day:

Breakfast:
1 cup cooked oatmeal 2 carbohydrate servings
1 cup low-fat Greek vanilla yogurt
1 dairy serving
1 cup blueberries
1 fruit serving
1 cup green tea beverage of choice

Morning Snack:
1 oz. low-fat string cheese
1 dairy serving
1 apple
1 fruit serving

Lunch:
3 oz. water-packed tuna
3 oz. protein
1 hard-boiled egg
1 oz. protein
Big green salad w/lots of veggies Unlimited
2 tsps. of olive oil
2 tsp. of added fat
Balsamic vinegar Unlimited
1 large whole-grain roll 2 carbohydrate servings

Afternoon Snack:
1 cup low-fat strawberry Greek yogurt
1 dairy serving
1 small banana
1 fruit serving

Dinner:
1½ cups of cooked brown rice
3 carbohydrate servings
5 oz. grilled chicken or fish
5 oz. protein
Steamed broccoli and carrots Unlimited
Drizzle of 3 tsps. olive oil on chicken or veggies 3 tsp. of added fat

Dessert:
1 cup of mixed berries w/spritz of whipped cream
1 fruit serving

If you tally up the servings, they come out to exactly the same numbers from the 2,100-calorie serving chart. Or if you wish to just loosely follow a sample menu plan in the appendix, it is all balanced out. Don't walk around with a calculator and drive yourself crazy. Just be aware of what you need in general and try to get it in as best you can. For most dancers, that means smaller meals or snacks to fit into crazy dance schedules.

Taking it to the Next Level

For those of you wishing to determine your basal metabolic rate more specifically so you know how many calories you deserve each day, you can use the formulas in the appendix. This is only if you wish to be more specific. However, remember that following the chart and calorie ranges loosely is also a good guide to a proper calorie intake.

On a final note, don't get hung up with calculations and being perfect. If you feel that you are not consuming anywhere near the recommended daily calories and are afraid to eat more, just notice:

• Could your energy be better?

• Could your mood improve?

• Do you get really hungry at night and crave sugar?

• Does being hungry interfere with your sleep?

• Are you experiencing muscle fatigue or having stamina issues?

• Are you getting injured or sustaining stress fractures?

Just start slowly by adding perhaps a piece of fruit and an extra yogurt or glass of milk. Then when you make the connection between a bit more food and feeling better, you can slowly add more in until you reach a more useful calorie level.

Read on into the next chapters to get a better view of what is needed on a daily basis in a practical way.

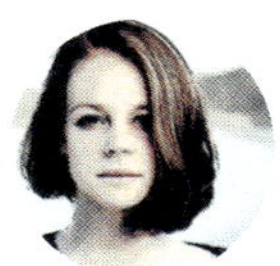

Callie wants to maintain her weight and her energy at the summer intensive. They are dancing everyone pretty hard all day. She now knows that dancers are elite athletes and deserve fuel! She wants to try to follow a sample 2,100-calorie menu in the appendix to feel if it is right for her. If she needs more food, she now knows she can add more and deserves more. Feeling hungry, light-headed, disoriented, getting sick all the time and feeling exhausted means she is not eating enough and hydrating enough. No dancer wants to feel that way! She will just plan ahead the night before and be prepared for the next day. By eating right, she will dance right!

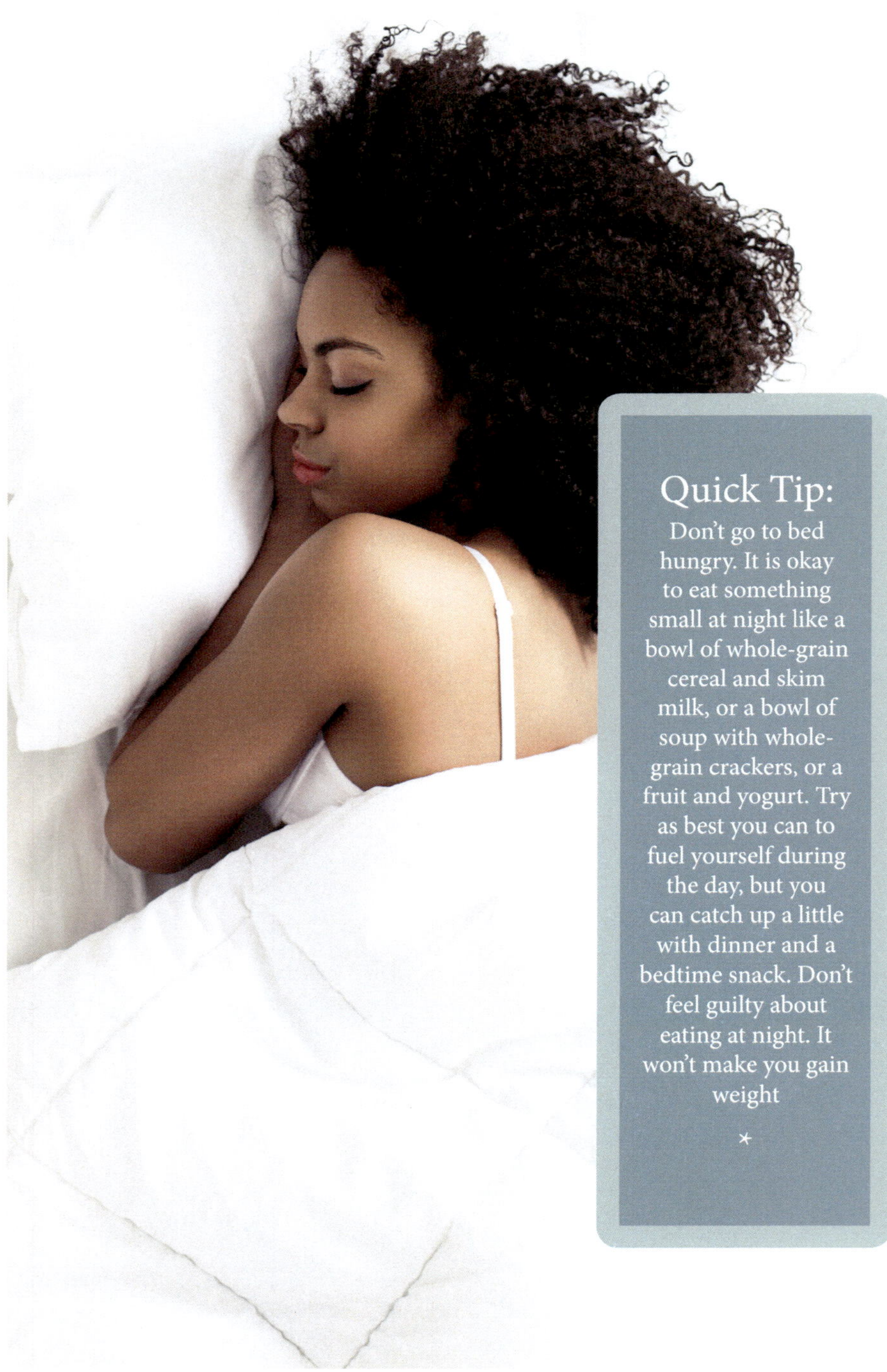

Quick Tip:

Don't go to bed hungry. It is okay to eat something small at night like a bowl of whole-grain cereal and skim milk, or a bowl of soup with whole-grain crackers, or a fruit and yogurt. Try as best you can to fuel yourself during the day, but you can catch up a little with dinner and a bedtime snack. Don't feel guilty about eating at night. It won't make you gain weight

★

Key Note: Feel it Out!

Once you get an idea of the number of calories you deserve, you can either go back to the calorie ranges and serving size chart earlier in the chapter, or you can go to the sample menus in the appendix and choose one to follow loosely around your calorie range. Make everything work for you. You may try to follow a plan and feel like you need a little more of something. Just add it in! Nutrition is not just a numbers game. You have to feel if it is right for your body. Eating healthfully means you have plenty of energy, stamina and endurance for your dance day with no crashes, sugar cravings, or generally feeling terrible.

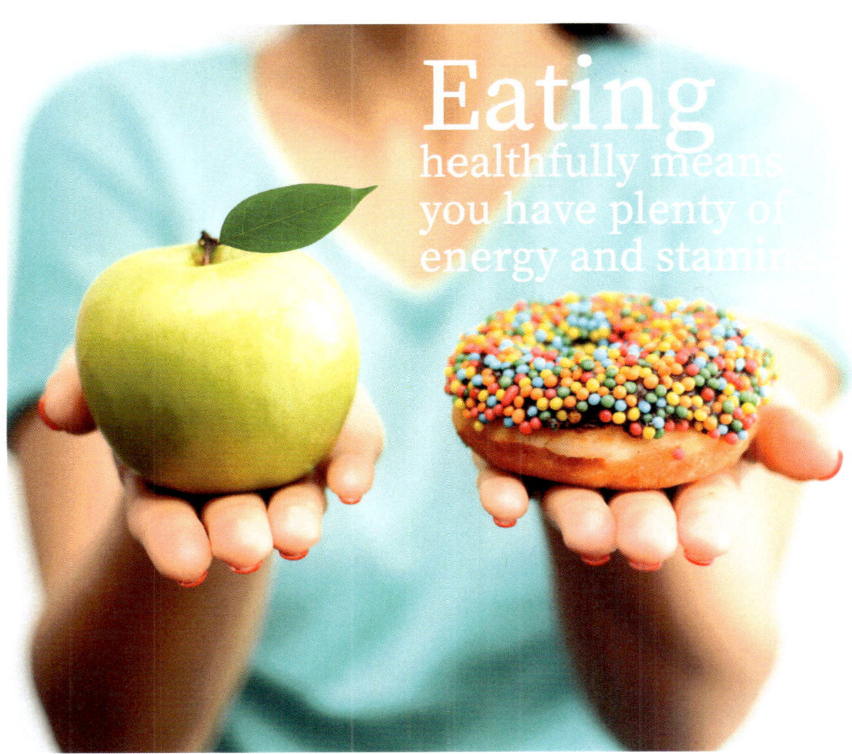

Review: Chapter 1

1.

Dancers need calories. Eating too few calories will seriously impair performance, mental alertness and may make you prone to injury by promoting muscle loss.

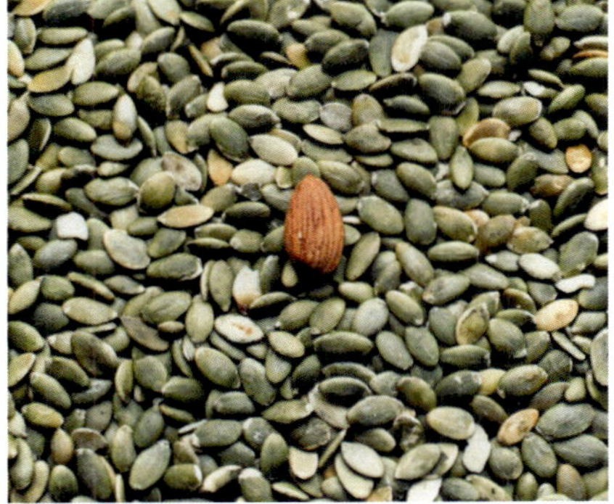

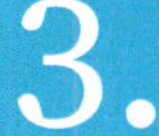

2.

Start early. Don't leave home without breakfast! Even if you don't like eating in the morning, have something like a small fruit and/or a low-fat Greek yogurt.

3.

Always combine good-quality protein with good-quality carbohydrates and some fat. An example for breakfast would be a cup of whole-grain oatmeal (carbohydrate) with a low-fat Greek yogurt (protein) and a handful of almonds (protein and good fat). This combination of all three macronutrients will keep you full longer, keep your blood sugar even and give you energy, and will keep you mentally alert. Also use the MyPlate visual in the appendix as a guide.

4.

Choose healthy foods from whole grains, lean proteins and good fats and greatly reduce "empty calories" from sugary sweets and refined flour products like cookies, pastries, and candy.

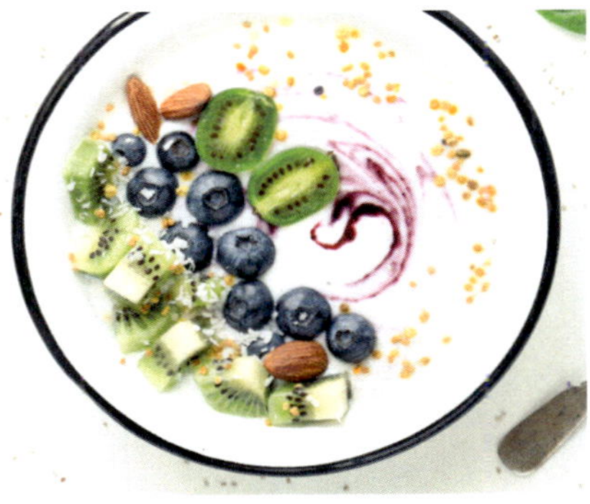

5.

This doesn't mean that you cannot have those fun foods; we just want to keep them limited, so they don't crowd out the healthier foods containing the nutrients you need for health.

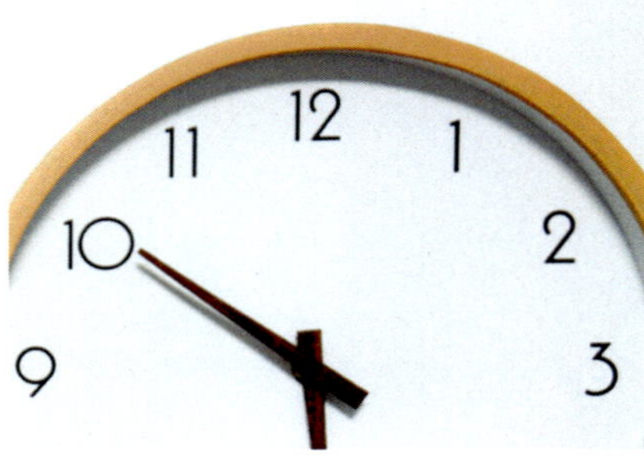

6.

Eat every four to five hours and snack often. Plan ahead. Anything liquid (like a protein and yogurt smoothie) will go down easily, not make you feel too full, and you can dance easily within twenty to thirty minutes after you consume it. So bring a thermos filled with a yogurt and banana shake and sip through busy dance times. It will keep you going until your next eating opportunity. Or you can munch on a peanut butter and jelly sandwich with a carton of soy milk and a piece of fruit throughout the afternoon, thereby keeping those calories in and energy high.

7.

If you do not eat all the calories you deserve, you will lose energy, lose mental focus, and crave sugar! You might even lose muscle!

8.

Don't follow fads or Hollywood celebrities. What is right for someone else may hurt your health and career. Pay attention to what YOU need and forget the rest. There are many "dietary" strategies out there, such as being vegan or vegetarian, or gluten-free or "raw." These eating options are not right for everyone. The best eating plan makes you feel good and is balanced with nutrients so that you don't have to rely on supplements to give you what your restrictive eating plan is missing. If you choose to be vegan or vegetarian, I suggest that you see a registered dietitian to make sure your food choices are healthy and balanced. I have included some vegan, vegetarian, and gluten-free menus in the appendix for your information if you need suggestions.

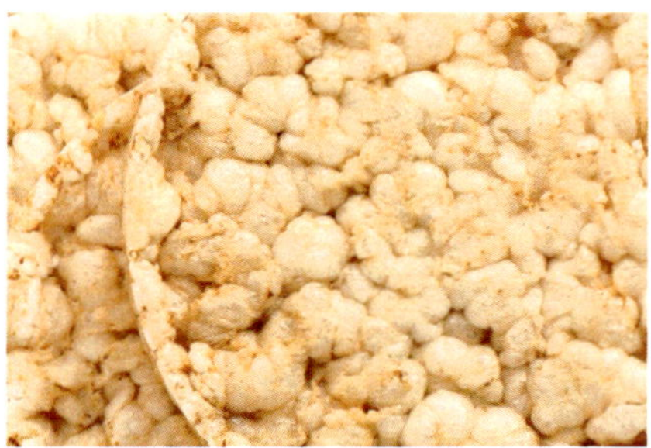

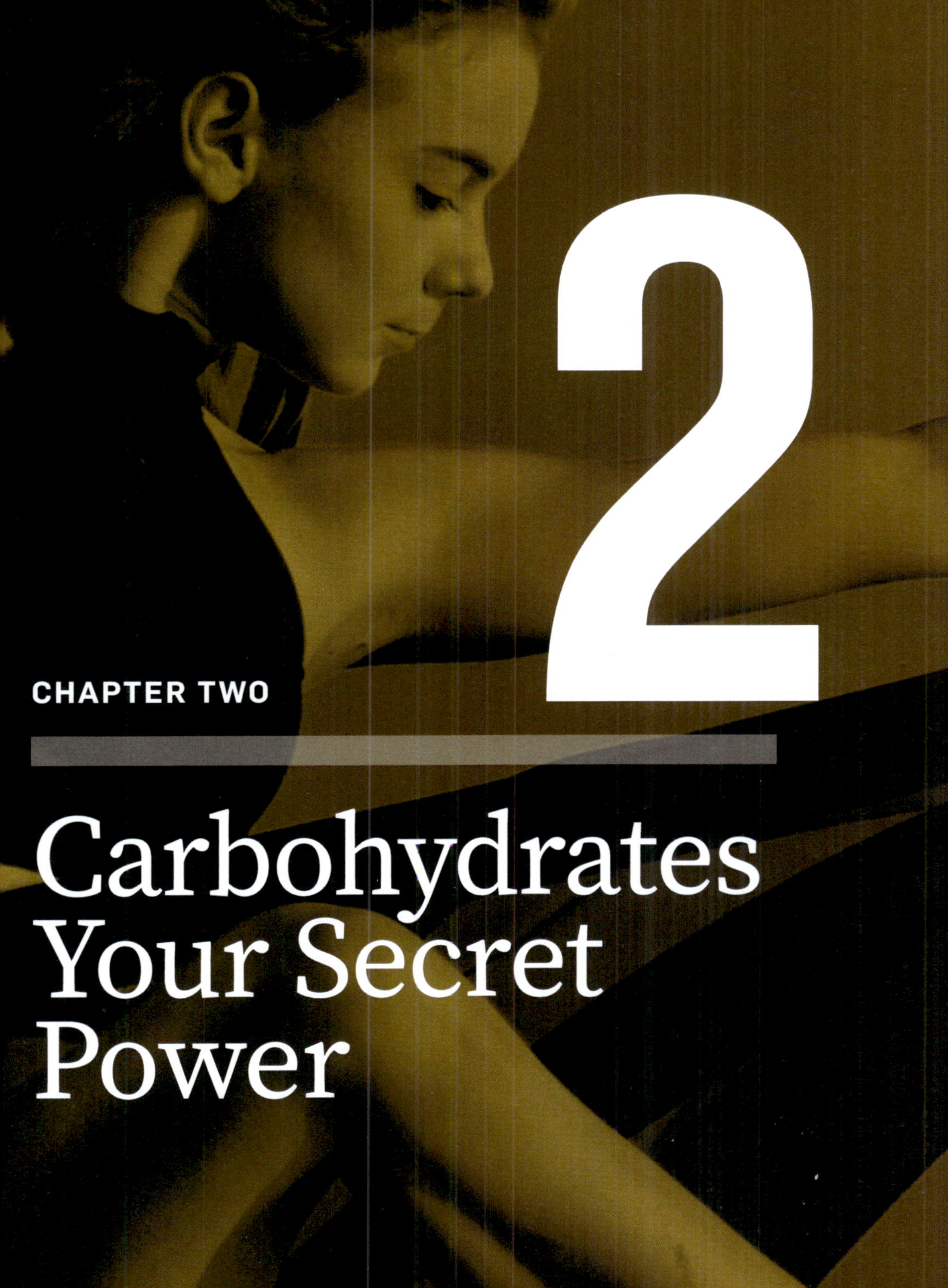

CHAPTER TWO
2
Carbohydrates
Your Secret
Power

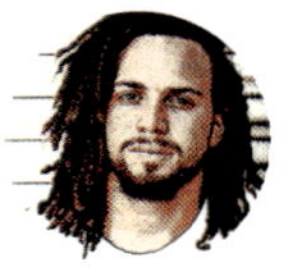

Gregory was told that carbohydrates would make him fat. He is worried about including them in his diet. He knows, though, that when he doesn't eat bread, cereals, grains, and potatoes, that his energy crashes, and he craves sugar! Have you ever been told that you should never eat bread, or that carbohydrates will make you gain weight, or that they create toxins? Here is the most important news you could ever hear: carbohydrates are the dancer's "secret" power.

> ## Fast Facts:
>
> Carbohydrates are the most powerful nutrient for your energy level. Carbohydrates provide you with the ability to dance with endurance and stamina.
> For all dancers, 50%–60% of each day's total calorie intake should be comprised of carbohydrates. Carbohydrates fuel the brain—without them, you cannot be mentally alert.
>
> *

Why? Because carbohydrates are the ONLY foods that can be digested quickly to deliver blood sugar to the brain, nervous system, and working muscles without creating metabolic distress. They keep you alert, mentally and physically focused, and ready to dance.

If you eliminate carbohydrates, you will

1. Crave sugar.

2. Will not get the vitamins and minerals you need for energy production and healthy immune system.

3. Will break down muscle to make blood sugar, thereby weakening joints, weakening your immune system, and lowering your metabolism.

The Dancer's Fuel: Here Is How It Works

The importance of carbohydrates in athletic and dance performance has been clearly established in scientific research. Unfortunately, as dancers, we are often taught that carbohydrates are the first foods to be eliminated when you try to lose weight. Eliminating carbohydrates is not the healthiest way to lose weight, if you need to, because this promotes loss of muscle, not fat. See chapter on "diets." When we talk about carbohydrates, we are mainly talking about plant foods, such as grains, potatoes, cereals, and foods made from grains such as breads and crackers, and fruits and vegetables. Here they are in chart form:

Type of Carbohydrate	What Is Included
Complex (Healthy)	Whole grains, oats, barley, quinoa, millet, spelt, whole-grain breads, cereals, pastas, potatoes, rice, whole fruits, and vegetables.
Simple (Not so healthy) Okay for a once in a while treat.	Sugar, high-fructose corn syrup, honey, molasses, and foods like donuts, cakes, cookies, pies, candy.
Fiber (Healthy)	Fiber is the indigestible part of the plant that keeps us full, keeps our blood sugar even, and helps us remove toxins and cholesterol from the body. Fiber is found only in whole foods like complex carbohydrates.

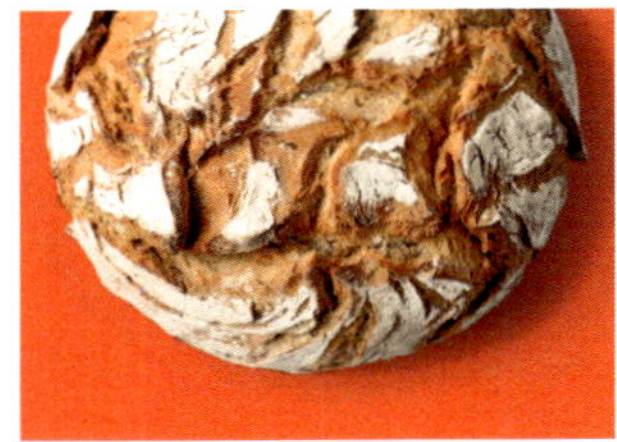

Complex carbohydrates are whole foods that contain all their naturally occurring vitamins, minerals, antioxidants, and fiber.

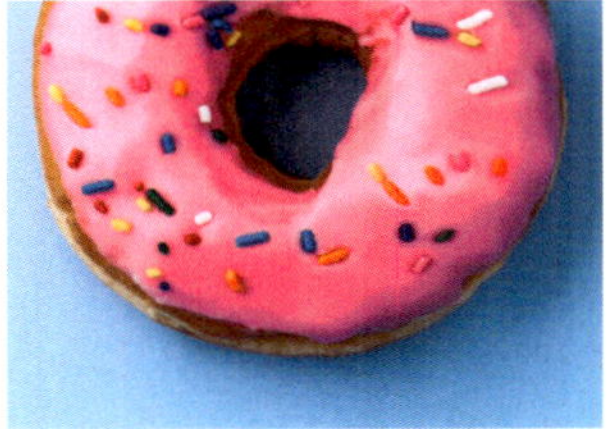

Simple carbohydrates are foods that have been refined, and the flour has been milled so that many vitamins, minerals, and fiber do not remain.

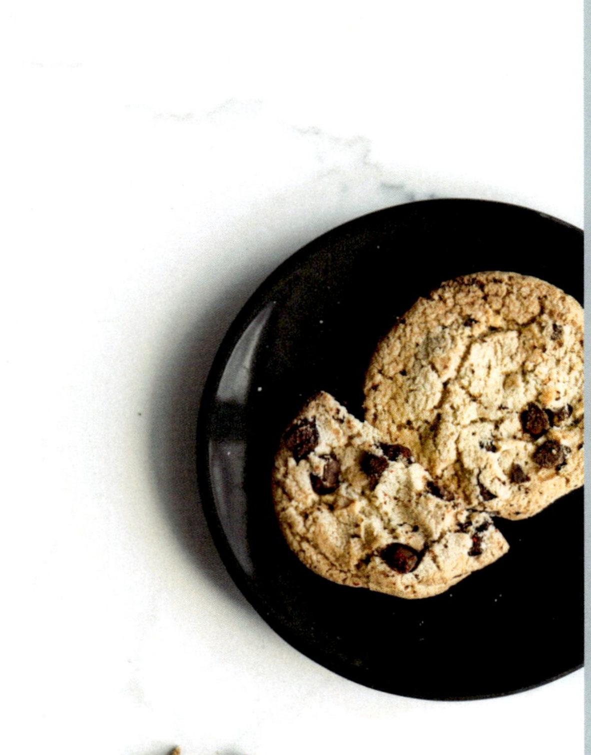

Fast Facts:

There is a place for simple carbohydrates and a bit of sugar in every dancer's diet! The "recommended" serving for something sweet is about 5% or less of our total calories. (World Health Organization) For most dancers that is about 100–200 calories from a sweet snack such as a square of chocolate, one or two of your favorite cookies with a cup of tea or have a half cup of frozen yogurt for a treat. There is nothing wrong if you like a bit of sweet! Having a bit of sugar often can make you feel like you are not in "food prison." Just don't have a box of cookies for breakfast!

*

A dancer's body is like a finely tuned machine. The gasoline that makes this machine work is carbohydrates. When we eat, say, a baked potato; that potato is broken down in digestion and transformed into glucose (or blood sugar). Because we need so much blood sugar each day to live and dance, the body has a way to store this blood sugar in our working muscles or liver. The storage form of blood sugar is called glycogen. We have the ability to store this glycogen, so we can have it for when we need it—like when we are dancing or active for long periods of time. It is these stored carbohydrate calories that determine how long you can dance and how mentally and physically focused you will be. The easiest way to know how much you need would be to just follow a sample menu plan that looks good to you. They are located in the appendix section of this guidebook. Just make it easy for yourself. Please note that we cannot store much glycogen, so we need to replenish these stores on a daily basis by eating cereals, breads, grains, potatoes, pastas, fruits, and vegetables. You must choose all three types of carbohydrates and eat all three categories every day. A bowl of broccoli cannot be substituted for a bowl of rice.

KEY NOTE FROM GREGORY:

Gregory has learned that if you are on a low-carbohydrate "diet" your muscles will be chronically fatigued, and you will be more prone to injury. Carbohydrates are used in the body twenty-four hours per day, seven days a week. Carbohydrates are also needed to fuel the brain and central nervous system. If carbohydrates are not eaten, we cannot live! If we do not consume this important food group, the only way we can survive is to break down protein including our own muscle to provide fuel. As a dancer, you do not want to lose muscle. To avoid this, 50%–60% of your daily calories should come from your starchy carbohydrates (pastas, potatoes, grains, cereals, breads) and fruits and veggies. Check out the calorie range chart in chapter 1 and the appendix for menu plans to see how much of every type of carbohydrate you need each day. Gregory had no idea that the key to building muscle and not breaking it down was to eat good-quality carbohydrates.

If you choose your calorie range as shown in the last chapter and loosely follow the serving sizes, you will automatically be consuming the appropriate balance of complex carbohydrates.

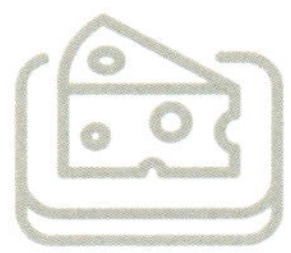
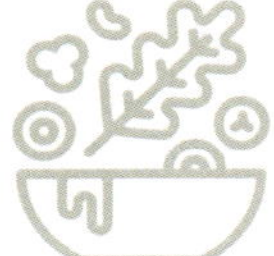
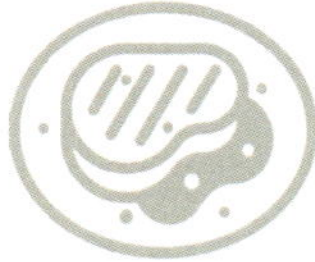
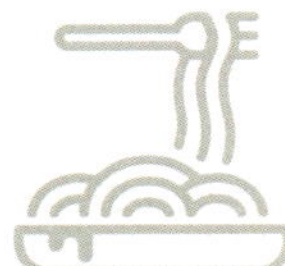

MyPlate: cover half your plate with veggies and one quarter of it with a grain, potato, pasta or bread. The other quarter of the plate will have your protein. Have fruit as part of breakfast or for a snack or healthy dessert. If you follow the visual of the plate, you will be eating in a balanced way for dance and life. See the appendix for your MyPlate picture.

Taking It to the Next Level:

See appendix I to determine specific grams of carbohydrates

KEY NOTE FROM GREGORY:

Gregory was trying to build muscle by downing protein shakes and filling up on burgers and eggs. All this did was to make him tired and actually unable to build muscle. By incorporating more good-quality carbohydrates, like oatmeal, sweet potatoes, brown rice and whole-grain pasta, he had the energy to do his weight training properly. Eating adequate but not excessive protein helps rebuild muscle mass without that protein having to be made into an energy source. Eating carbohydrates allows protein to be used to repair muscle and not used to make blood sugar. So now, Gregory is gaining the upper body strength that he needs for partnering and dance in general! And his energy is going through the roof!

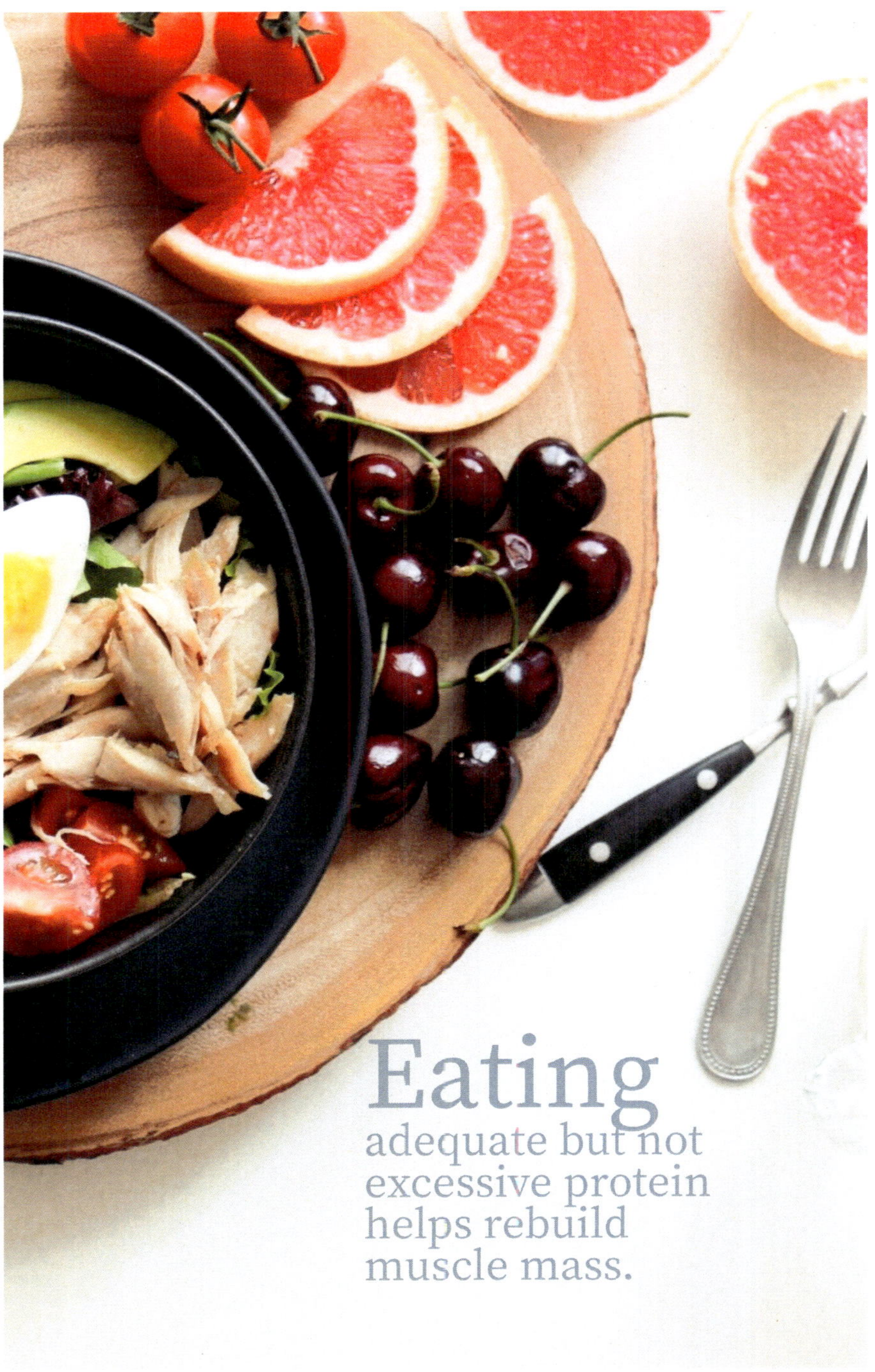

Eating
adequate but not
excessive protein
helps rebuild
muscle mass.

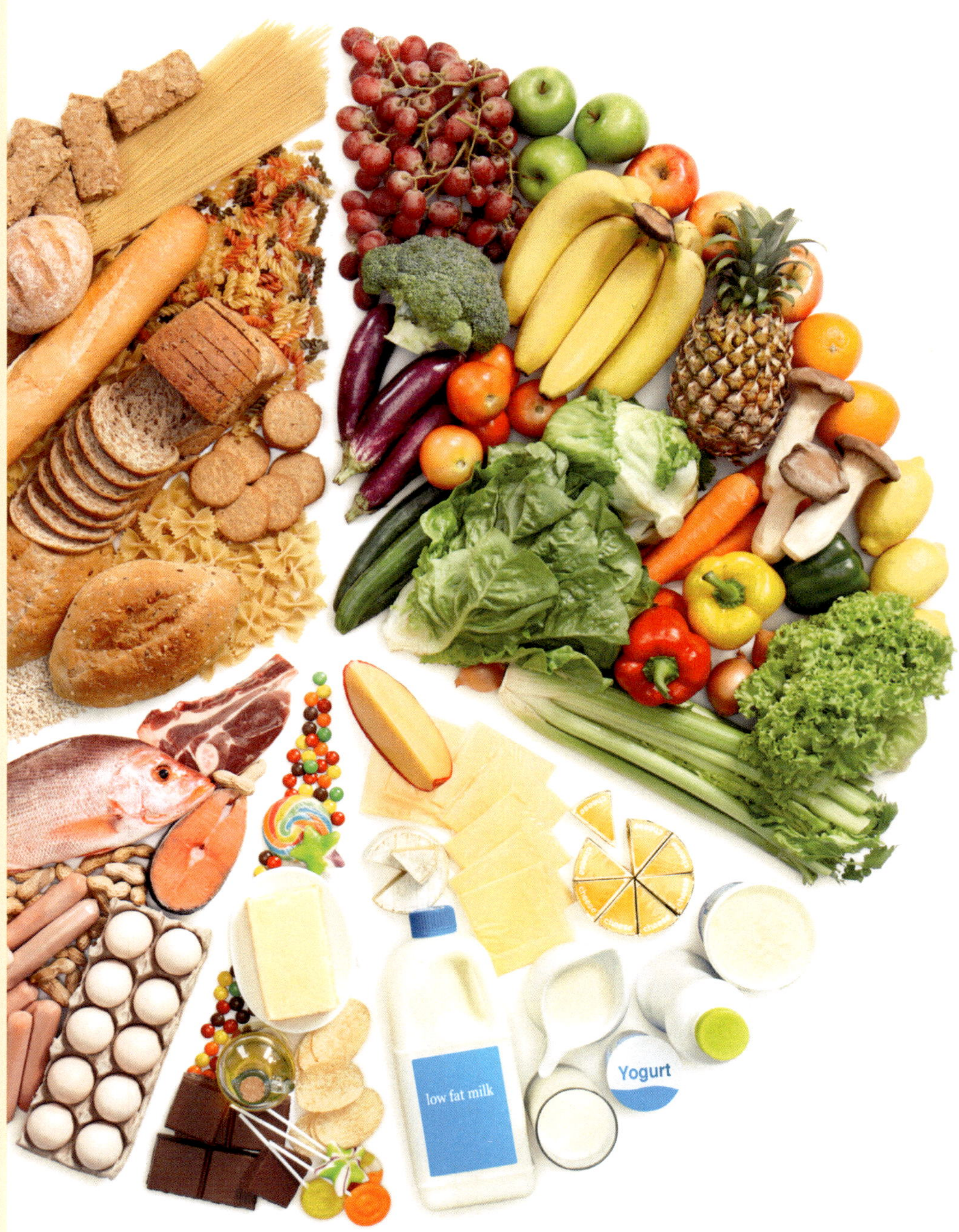

low fat milk
Yogurt

Get a general idea of where your carbohydrates come from

Bread, Cereal, Grain, Potato Group
Examples of one serving are:
1. 1 slice of bread (check labels)
2. ½ cup cooked grain like rice, cereal, pasta, or mashed potato
3. ½ cup corn or peas
4. 1/3 baked potato
5. 1/8 bagel
6. 15 french fries

One serving is:
1. 80 calories or one ounce and = 15 grams of carbohydrates

Fruit Group
Examples of one serving are:
1. 1 small fruit
2. ¾ cup fruit juice
3. ¼ cup dried fruit
4. ½ cup chopped fresh fruit
5. 15 grapes

One serving is:
1. 60 calories = 15 grams of carbohydrates

Vegetable Group
Examples of one serving are:
1. ½ cup cooked or chopped raw
2. 1 cup leafy greens

One serving is:
1. 25 calories = 5 grams of carbohydrates

Dairy Group
Dairy foods are mostly protein, but they do contribute carbohydrates from milk sugar
Examples of one serving are:
1. 1 cup milk, yogurt, soy or almond milk
2. 1 oz. cheese
3. ¼ cup cottage cheese

One serving is:
1. 80–150 calories = 12 grams of carbohydrate which comes from the natural sugars in milk

Sports nutrition studies tell us that most dancers and athletes should consume between 6–10 grams of carbohydrates per kilogram of body weight (take weight in pounds and divide by 2.2 to get kilograms of body weight). That pans out to between 200–300 grams of carbohydrates daily approximately.

All in a Dancer's Day: The trick is for dancers to eat 4–5 times per day with a little carbohydrate at each meal and snack. This will provide you with consistent energy, help keep you focused, and keep sugar cravings low. That's a good thing and what a dancer wants. Gregory has learned the hard way that good-quality whole grains, cereals, breads, fruits and veggies will keep him going all day in New York. He has goals to achieve and wants to land his first job on Broadway giving it his all. He cannot do that if his diet is not balanced. He is going to include oatmeal, brown rice, and sweet potatoes every day! Snacks will be fresh fruit, and he will make lunch a salad base with carbohydrates, protein, and fat to round it out. Broadway, watch out!

And Remember: Carbohydrates are indeed your "secret" power. Never eliminate them totally if you want to dance well or dance at all.

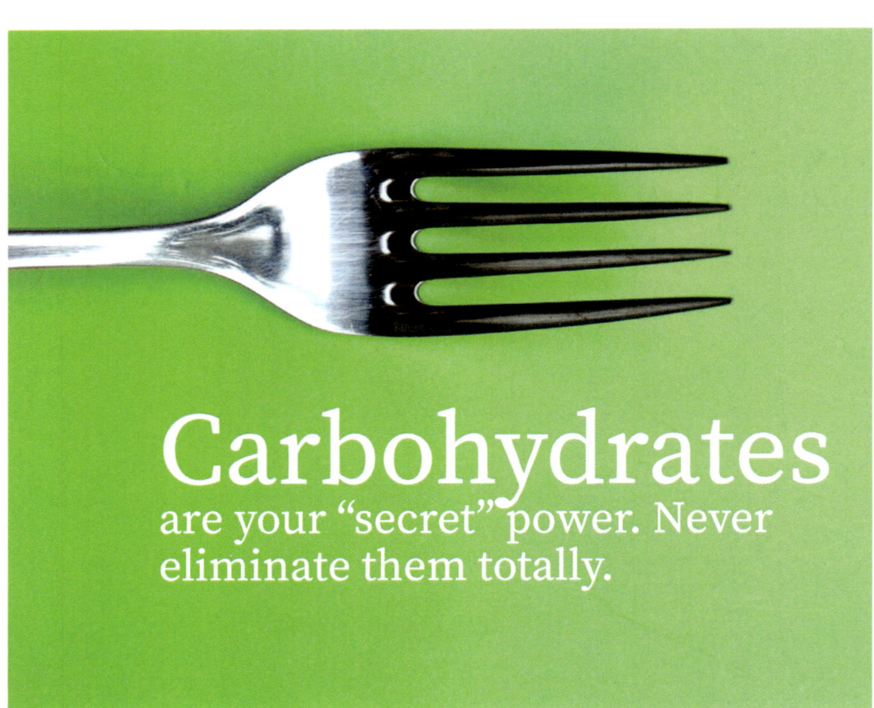

Fast Facts:

Take note of the great nutrients you will miss if you eliminate carbohydrates:

Nutrient	Importance	Good Sources
Potassium	Prevents muscle cramps and promotes good heart function	Peaches, pears, cantaloupe, squash, potatoes, asparagus, tomatoes
Magnesium	Keeps bones healthy, needed for the release of energy in the body	Spinach, seaweed, zucchini, sesame and sunflower seeds, beets, turnip greens, broccoli, bok choy
Iron	Needed for energy, carries hemoglobin in the blood, which carries oxygen to your muscles	Spinach, prunes, raisins, dried apricots, dates, figs, lima beans, parsley
Vitamin C	Needed for immunity and to make collagen for healthy joints	Citrus fruits, cantaloupe, broccoli, green peppers, strawberries, papaya, mango
B Vitamins	Important for energy production, cell protection, and healthy digestive system	Fortified cereals, breads, grains, peas, beans, lettuce, mushrooms, mustard greens
Vitamin K	For good digestion, for immunity, for blood clotting factors	Leafy green vegetables
Vitamin A	Promotes good night vision, helps the thyroid gland to work, helps manufacture red blood cells, and helps the adrenal glands	Carrots, sweet potatoes, spinach, greens, butternut squash
Fiber	Promotes healthy digestion, removes cholesterol and toxins from our bodies and helps keep us full and satisfied. Essential for maintaining optimal weight and for healthy weight loss	Whole grains, cereals, breads, whole-grain pastas, potatoes, whole fruits and vegetables

Review: Chapter 2

1.

Always fill one quarter of your plate with a complex carbohydrate (cereals, grains, potatoes, pasta, whole-grain breads/crackers).

3.

Choose brown rice, whole wheat pasta, white and sweet potatoes, and other grains like millet, couscous, and wild rice.

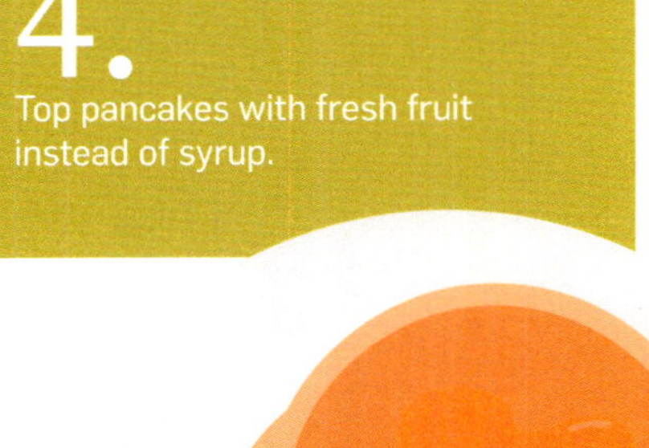

4.

Top pancakes with fresh fruit instead of syrup.

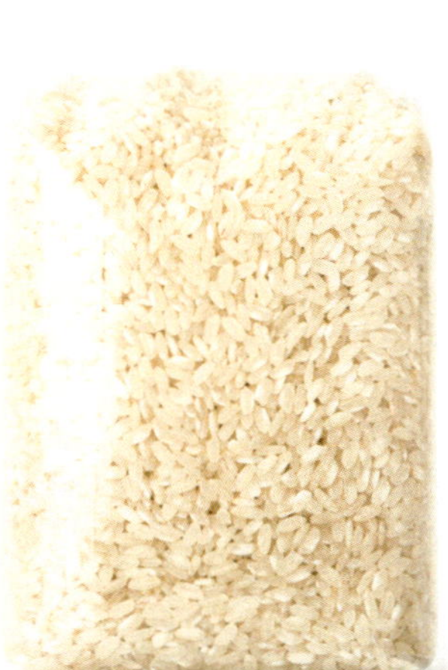

2.

Try whole-grain cereals, oatmeal, buckwheat pancakes, whole-grain flour tortillas and whole-grain crackers.

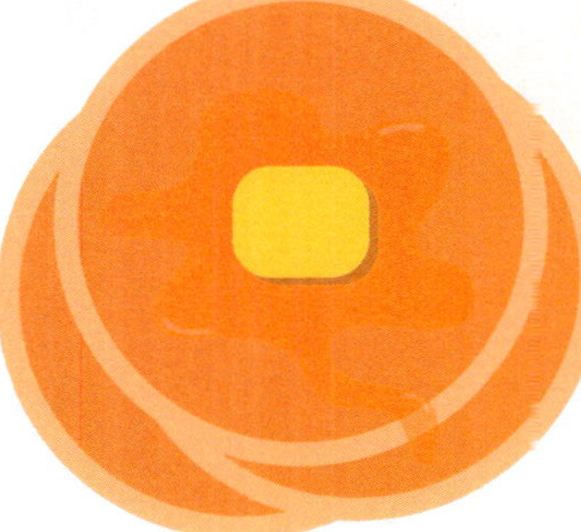

5.

Add fresh or dried fruit to homemade baked products or cereal

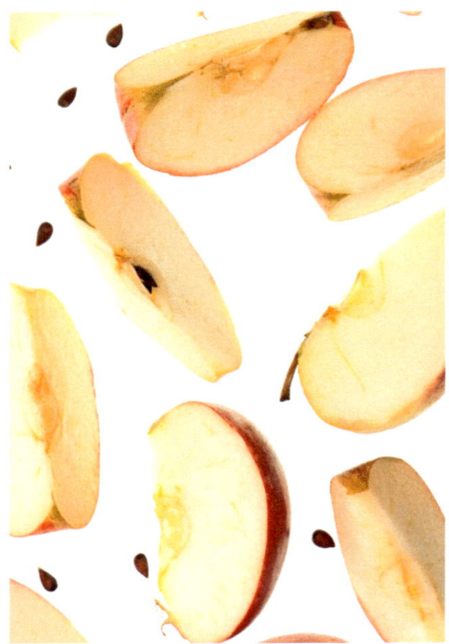

6.

Consume low-fat or nonfat dairy products. Try soy milk or almond milk if allergic to regular milk

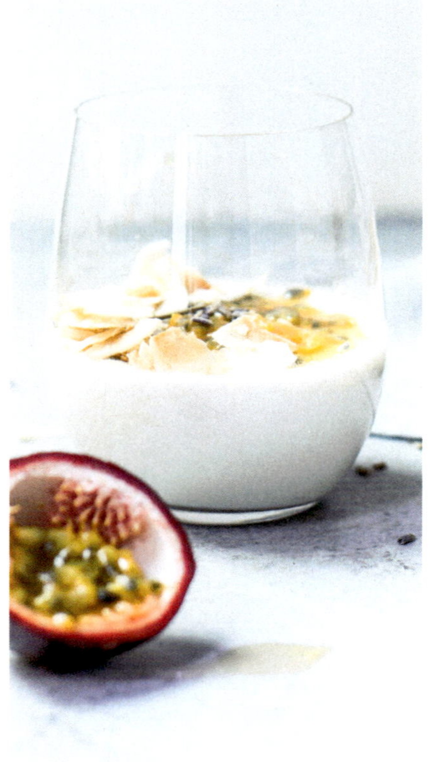

7.

Have a sweet snack of about 100–200 calories a few times a week. It will make you happy and not wreck your health. A little refined sugar is okay if 80% of the time we are eating wholesome, unprocessed foods.

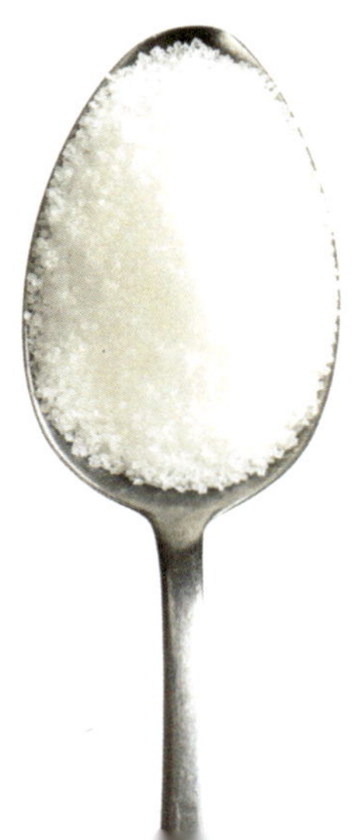

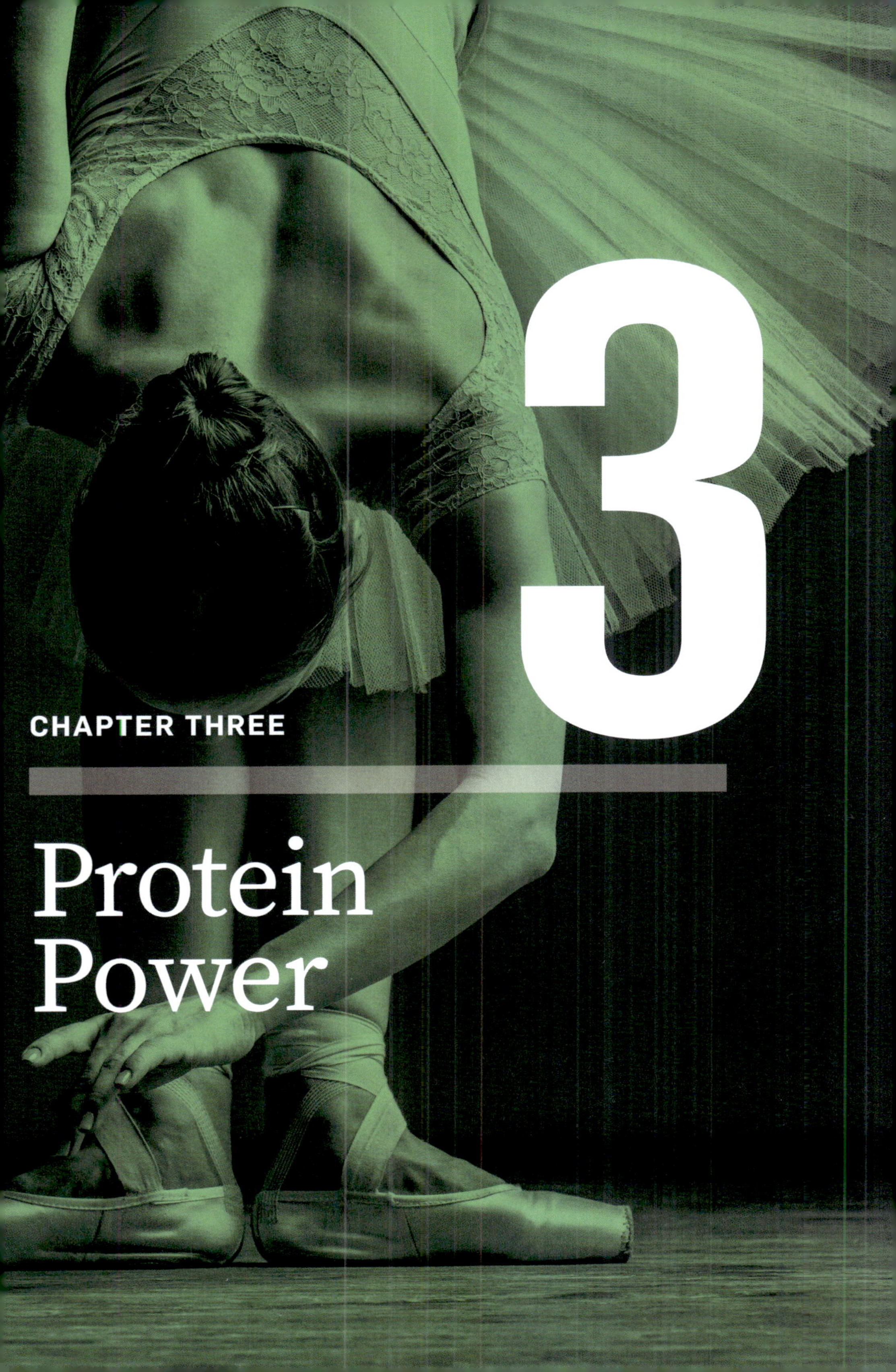
3
CHAPTER THREE
Protein
Power

Callie and Gregory have heard that high-protein diets are healthy, especially for dancers. Some of the dancers at Callie's intensive are following some of the popular high-protein diets and think that this is healthy. Some of Gregory's friends are just eating salad and chicken all day and wondering why they are exhausted. What is true and what is right for them, and you?

Here are some interesting facts: Approximately 75% of skeletal muscle is water! Only 20% of skeletal muscle is protein, and the remaining 5% is made up of inorganic salts, nutrients, and other substances. In the dance world, you may hear that eating more protein is better for you because people believe that carbohydrates make you gain weight, but this is not necessarily the truth. People gain weight generally because they consume too many calories from all foods and do not exercise!

We need protein to:

1. help build and repair muscle,
2. to help make hormones and red and white blood cells, and
3. to provide iron to help carry oxygen in our bodies for energy.
4. maintain the pH balance in our bodies and to keep fluids balanced.

The role of protein in food is not to provide the body with proteins directly but to supply the amino acids it contains so that our bodies can make its own proteins. There are 22 amino acids the body uses. Some amino acids can be made in the body. However, there are some amino acids that the body cannot make for itself, so they must be provided by our food. These are called essential amino acids, and they are isoleucine, histidine, leucine, lysine, methionine, phenylalanine, threonine, tryptophan, and valine.

What we call a "complete" protein contains all of the amino acids essential in human nutrition in adequate amounts to be used by our bodies. As dancers and athletes, we want to focus on consuming "high-quality protein" daily. This is defined as an easily digestible "complete" protein whose amino acids fit the pattern needed by our bodies. See key note.

So what do dancers need on a daily basis? We talk about protein in terms of the number of grams of protein needed for health and energy on a daily basis. Your protein needs can be calculated by your weight (1.2–1.5 grams/kg) (divide your weight in pounds by 2.2 to get kilograms of weight) or calculated by percentage of your daily calories (15%–20%). On average, most female dancers need around 80 grams of protein daily. On average, most male dancers need about 100 grams of protein daily.

KEY NOTE:

So how do we get these complete proteins into our diets? First, we need to know where our protein comes from. Our most complete proteins come from lean meats, poultry like chicken and turkey, fish, eggs, soy, and our dairy foods such as milk, cheese and yogurt. We also get protein, although it is incomplete, from our carbohydrates like grains, breads, and cereals, from our vegetables, from legumes (beans and peas), from nuts and seeds. That means that these nonmeat proteins must be consumed with other foods that supply their missing amino acids. Another reason for a varied diet!

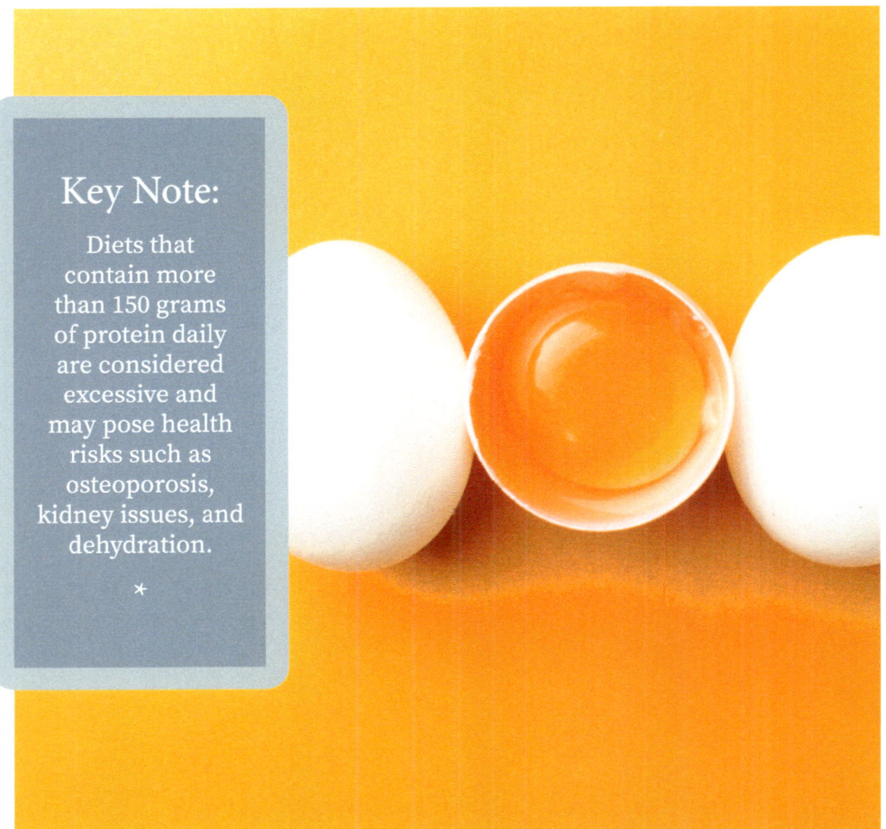

Key Note:

Diets that contain more than 150 grams of protein daily are considered excessive and may pose health risks such as osteoporosis, kidney issues, and dehydration.

*

Taking It to the Next Level:

See the appendix for calculating protein grams

A simple way of seeing how much protein you need is either to take a look at the calorie range chart in chapter 1 or see the appendix for protein calculations or the appendix with sample menu plans. For most female dancers that breaks down to 2–3 dairy servings and about 8 ounces of meat, fish, poultry, eggs, or the equivalent in soy, nuts and beans. For most male dancers that breaks down to 3–4 dairy servings and about 10 to 12 ounces of meat, fish, poultry, eggs, or the equivalent in soy, nuts and beans to be divided into 3–4 meals/snacks.

Here is a chart of protein sources:

Protein Sources	Yield
Lean red meat, chicken, turkey, fish	1 ounce = 7 grams of protein
Nonmeat sources like 1 egg, 2 egg whites, 2 tbsps. nut butter, 1/3 cup of nuts, 4 oz. tofu, ½ cup cooked beans	7 grams of protein
Dairy foods: 1 cup of milk or soy milk, 1 cup yogurt, 1 oz. cheese, ¼ cup cottage cheese	Approximately 7–8 grams of protein
Complex carbohydrates such as 1 slice bread, ½ cooked cereal, grain or pasta, 3 oz. potato, 80 calories worth of cereal	Approximately 3 grams of protein (incomplete - needs to be combined with other proteins to be used in the body)
Vegetables such as 1 cup leafy salad greens or ½ cup any cooked vegetable	Approximately 3 grams of protein (incomplete - needs to be combined with other proteins to be used in the body)

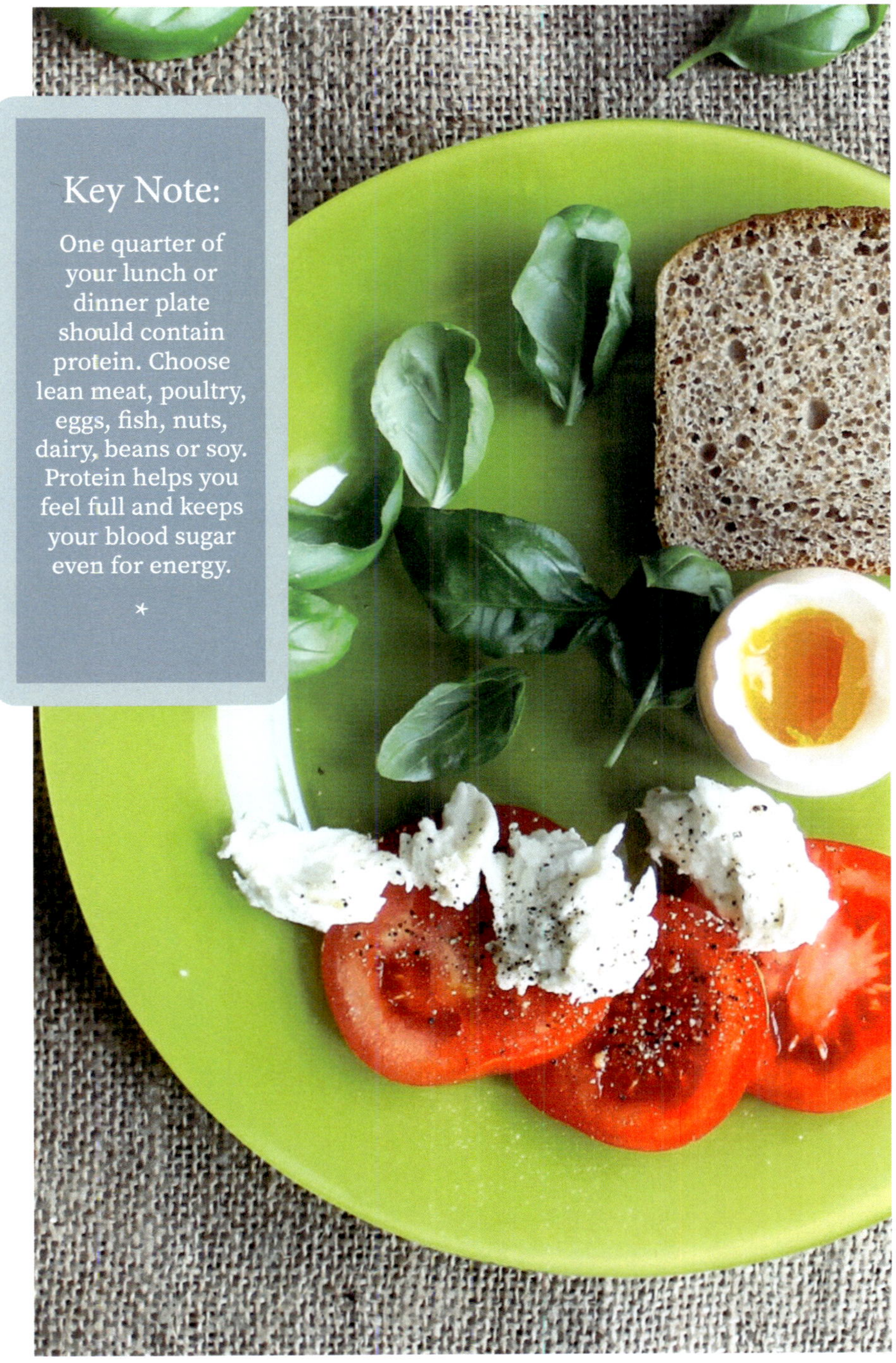

Key Note:

One quarter of your lunch or dinner plate should contain protein. Choose lean meat, poultry, eggs, fish, nuts, dairy, beans or soy. Protein helps you feel full and keeps your blood sugar even for energy.

*

More good news about protein*

Nutrient	Importance
Vitamin D	Needed for bone calcification.
Vitamin B1 (thiamine)	Needed to prevent the degeneration of nerves and muscles, loss of appetite, mental depression and neurological dysfunction.
Vitamin B2 (riboflavin)	Needed for metabolic reactions that release energy in cells. Also prevents lesions in the skin, eye, and mouth.
Vitamin B6 (pyridoxine)	There is usually no deficiency of this vitamin because it is available from these foods.
Pantothenic Acid	Needed for metabolism of carbohydrates, fats, and proteins and in the formation of cholesterol. Also prevents irritability, restlessness, fatigue, and leg cramps.
Folate	Needed for formation of normal red blood cells and of DNA and RNA. Also prevents anemia, prevents birth defects, and helps production of white blood cells.
B12	Needed for normal growth, maintenance of nerve tissue and for the formation of blood. Prevents pernicious anemia, sore tongue, weight loss, mental and nervous disorders, and degeneration of the spinal cord.
Magnesium	Needed for bone mineralization and for metabolism of carbohydrates, fats and protein. Needed for muscle function and the conduction of nerve impulses.
Calcium	Needed for bone mineralization, for maintaining normal function in muscles, for blood clotting and for the transport of fluid across cell membranes.
Phosphorus	An essential component of compounds crucial for energy production. Also helps to buffer acidity of the blood.
Iron	A structural component of hemoglobin, the oxygen-carrying compound in red blood cells.
Niacin	Needed for the release of energy from the breakdown of carbohydrates, proteins, and fats. Prevents dermatitis, diarrhea and depression.
Zinc	Needed for immune function, for wound healing, to prevent loss of taste and smell.

Good Sources

Fortified dairy foods

Lean red meats and poultry, dairy, nuts, fish, eggs, and beans

Lean red meats, poultry, fish, nuts, dairy foods, eggs, nuts and beans

Lean red meat, poultry, fish, dairy foods, eggs, nuts and beans

Egg yolks and liver

Lean red meats, poultry, fish, dairy foods, eggs, nuts and beans

Liver, kidney, eggs, and cheese. Also the body makes B12.

Dairy foods, poultry, fish, eggs, nuts and beans.

Dairy foods, fish, eggs, nuts and beans

Dairy foods, poultry, fish, nuts, eggs and beans

Lean red meat, poultry, fish, eggs, nuts and beans, dried fruit

Lean red meats, poultry, fish, nuts and beans

Lean red meats, fish, dairy foods, eggs, and beans

Healthier Proteins

1. Lean red meat like steak or roast beef
2. White meat poultry no skin
3. Fish
4. Beans
5. Nuts
6. Eggs and egg whites
7. Low-fat dairy foods
8. Soy in moderation

Not-So-Healthy Proteins

1. Luncheon meats or cold cuts
2. Bacon, sausage, or other fatty meats
3. Dark meat poultry with skin
4. High-fat dairy like cheeses should be consumed in moderation

Protein
helps you feel full and keeps your blood sugar even for energy.

*Take note of the nutrients you will miss if you are not consuming enough protein.

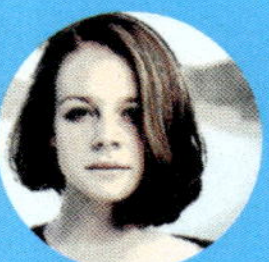

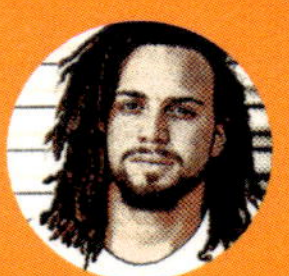

Don't go around with a calculator and try to tally your grams of protein. If you follow my serving size suggestions and calorie range chart, you will automatically be consuming adequate protein. Or just choose one of the menu plans in the appendix.

Even if you are trying to build muscle, you don't need a lot of extra protein! There is no scientific evidence that shows that consuming more than 2.0 grams of protein per kilogram of weight will help us build muscle. Proper resistance training with free weights or machines will help build muscle. You just have to consume enough calories, carbohydrates, proteins, and fats to increase your lean body mass. Training research suggests doing some resistance training three times per week and eating well should help build muscle SLOWLY over time. Be patient and don't overtrain.

Regularly scheduled rest days are critical for all dancers; otherwise, muscles and joints get too fatigued, and it is easy to injure yourself. So whether in dance class or the gym, try for variety in your routine and plan regularly scheduled rest days for muscles to repair and grow. Weight training may not be appropriate during a busy dance season. Train in the off season to reduce risk of injury.

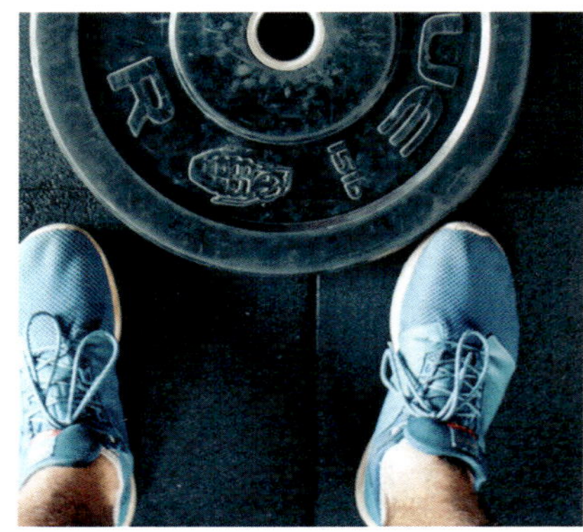

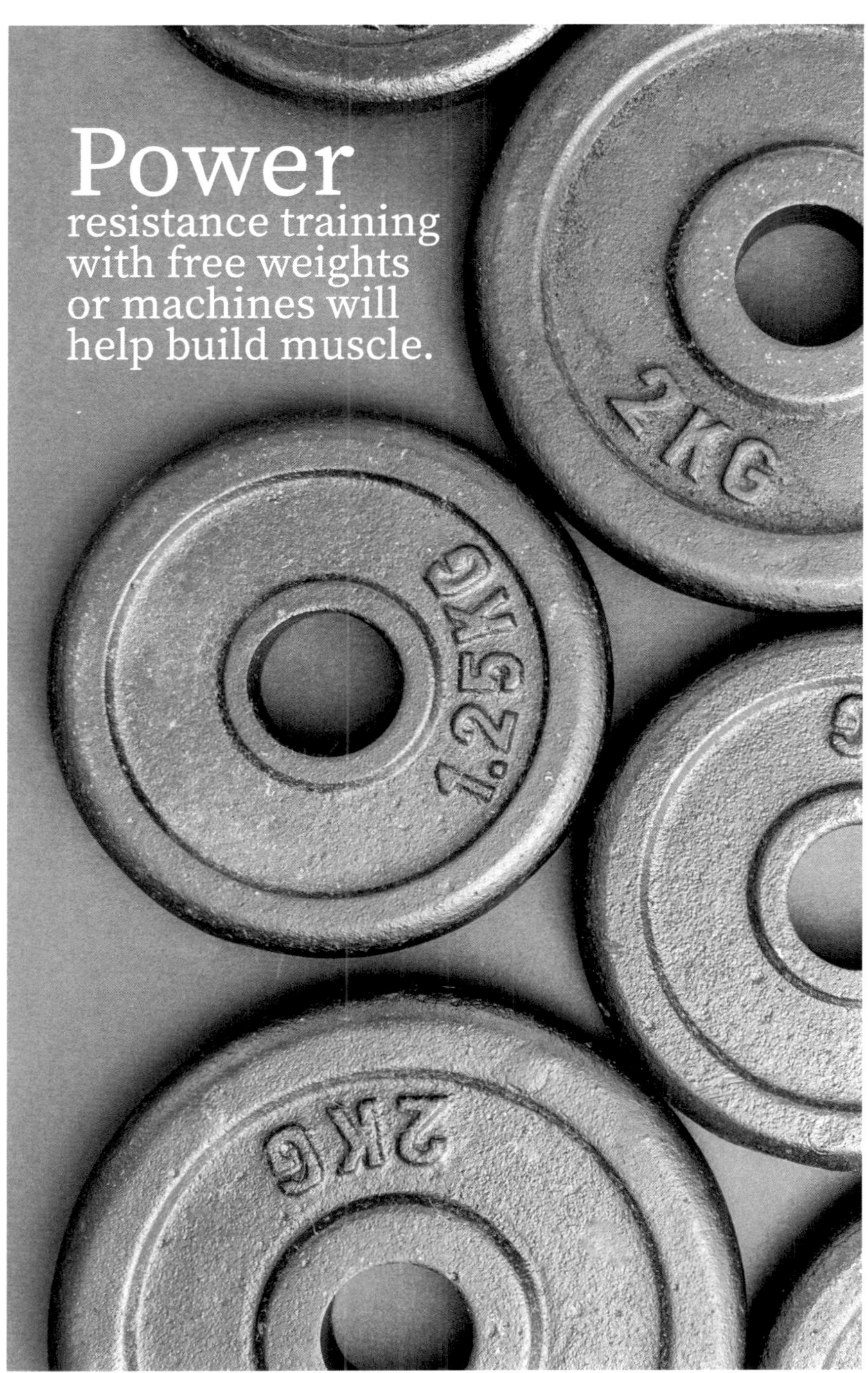

Power
resistance training
with free weights
or machines will
help build muscle.

Review: Chapter 3

1.

Adequate protein in our diets promotes a healthy immune system, helps us build and repair muscle, provides iron to prevent anemia and helps us maintain a proper fluid balance.

3.

Good sources of protein include lean red meat, poultry, fish, beans, nuts, eggs and egg whites, soy and dairy foods. Become a "flexitarian" and consume protein from plant and animal sources.

4.

Eliminating carbohydrates and eating a high-protein diet will actually promote muscle loss if enough calories are not consumed. It will also promote fluid loss, muscle cramps, headache, fatigue, joint inflammation, and may even contribute to bone loss.

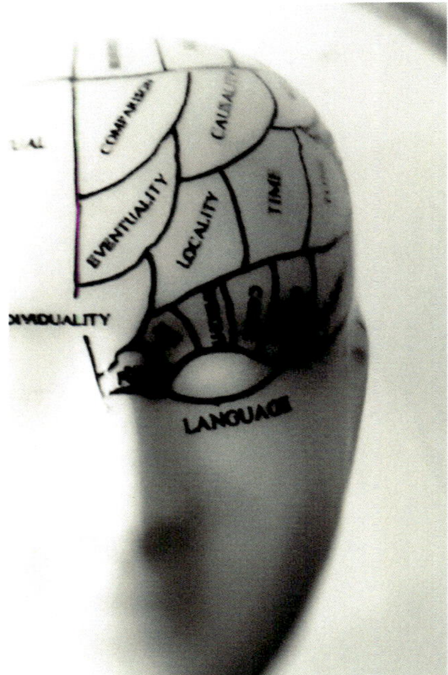

2.

Having protein at each meal and snack combined with a good-quality carbohydrate can help us keep our energy and blood sugar even, improve mental focus and keep us full and satisfied.

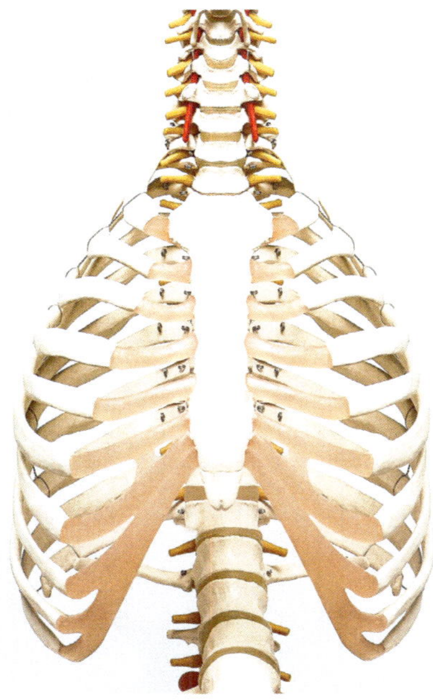

5.

Remember that you will also get some protein from your starchy carbohydrates and your veggies. It is difficult to NOT get enough protein in.

6.

Our bodies cannot absorb more than 30 grams of protein at any one time. That is the equivalent to approximately 5 oz. of protein. Downing protein shakes that contain more than 30 grams of protein at any one time just means you are wasting protein and wasting money.

7.

Don't get "hypnotized" by thinking you should follow what everyone else is doing. Get the facts! Don't follow a fad just to fit in. Doing so may compromise your ability to dance and can affect your health. Be smart about what is good for you and stick to "your" plan.

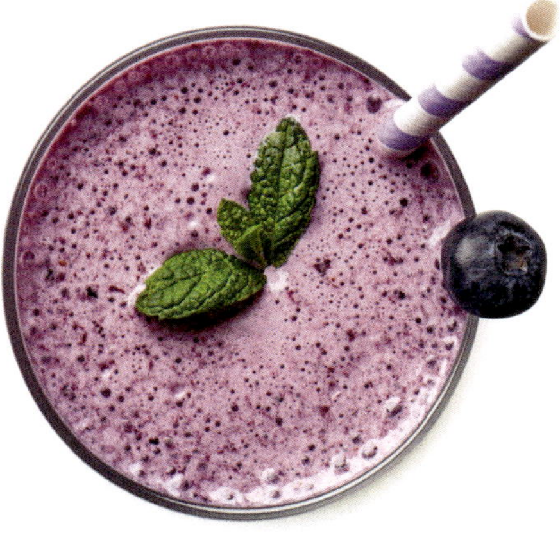

8.

It is especially important for vegans and vegetarians to have enough calories and varied food choices to make the complete proteins that their bodies need. If you have to rely on bars and protein powders to get enough protein in, it may be time to rethink your food choices so that you can stay healthy. See the appendix for some examples of vegan and vegetarian eating plans.

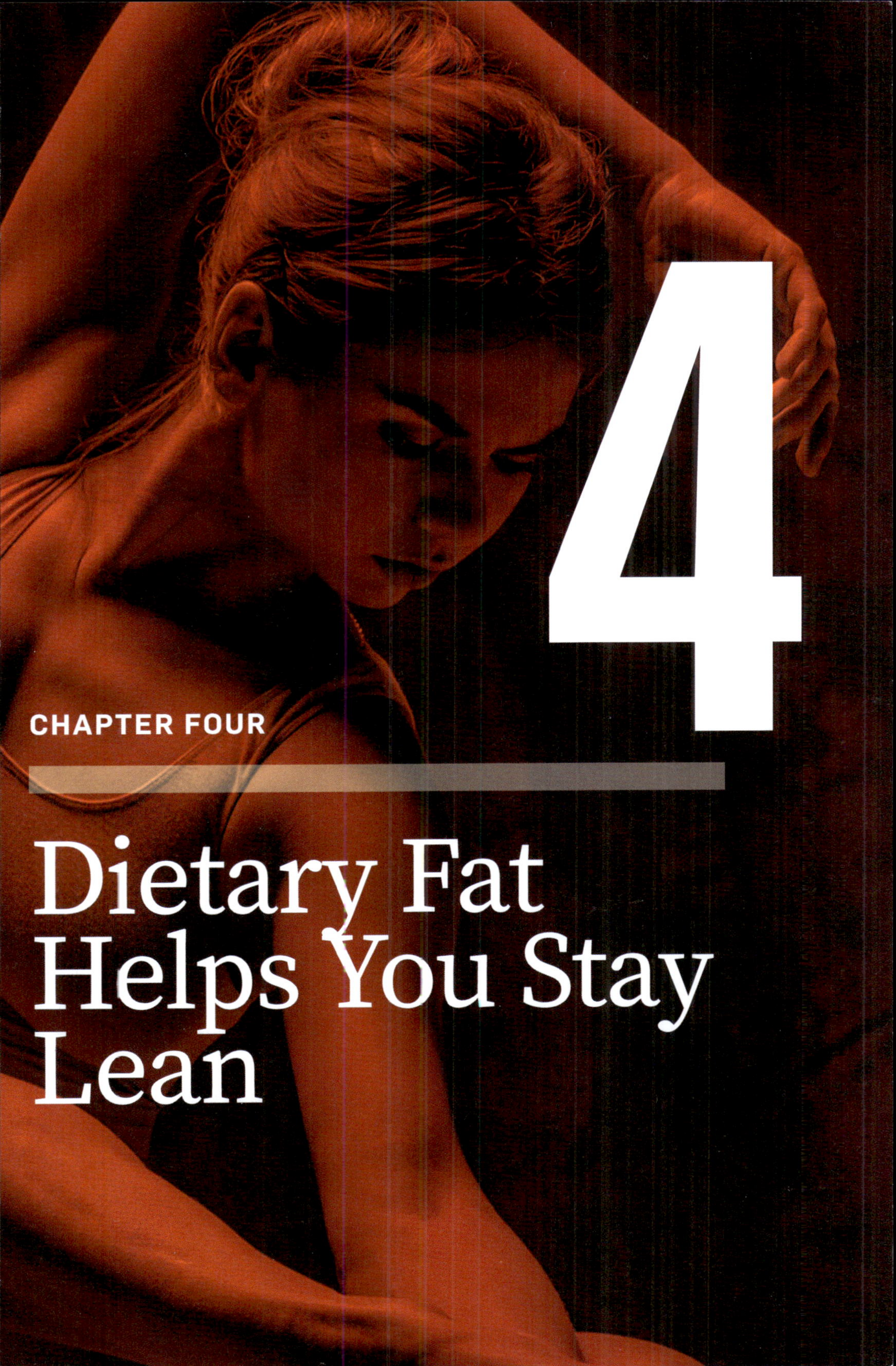

Dietary Fat Helps You Stay Lean

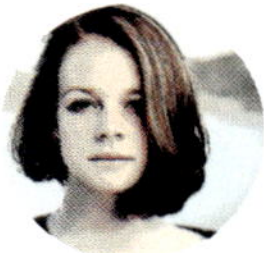

Fat's role in the body

Dietary fat serves many purposes in our bodies. It helps to maintain the structure and health of all cells. It provides essential fatty acids that are needed for a healthy immune function, healthy skin, healthy eyes and good brain function. These essential fats are fats that the body cannot make and must be supplied from our diets such as omega-3 fats and linoleic acid. (See chart for sources.)

Dietary fat helps us make hormones such as thyroid hormone, estrogen, progesterone, and testosterone. Dietary fat helps our bodies absorb fat-soluble vitamins like vitamins A, D, E, and K as well as antioxidants and phytonutrients. Consuming the right type of fat will also reduce inflammation, thereby protecting the dancer's joints and heart and lowering risk for developing rheumatoid arthritis. Fat also makes our foods taste delicious and helps us feel satisfied after eating, thereby preventing overeating. If we reduce fat too much in our diet, we will be hungry all the time and can make us feel unsatisfied! A little fat goes a long way in keeping us at a proper weight for our height.

Our body fat protects our body's organs from extremes in temperature and provides cushioning and protection from physical trauma. How much body fat should we have? For most women (nondancers), body fat within 21%–24% of weight is considered healthy. For most female dancers, body fat between

Consuming
the right type of fat will help reduce inflamation.

16%–21% seems the norm. If a woman's body fat falls below 12% of her weight, her health may be seriously compromised. This is not optimal. For most men (nondancers), body fat within 12%–16% of weight is considered healthy. For most male dancers, body fat between 7%–12% seems the norm. Male Olympic athletes can often get their body fat to 3%, but it would be dangerous and unhealthy to maintain this for any length of time for any male dancer. See your registered dietitian (RD) for a body fat percentage reading to get a sense of whether you are within a healthful range, not to berate yourself for not being thin enough. I guarantee that you will be surprised at how lean you are and how much muscle you have. One of the most accurate ways to measure body fat is to use what is called bioelectrical impedance. Handheld machines or the scales that you step on are wildly inaccurate. Your RD will be able to measure this and put it in perspective for you.

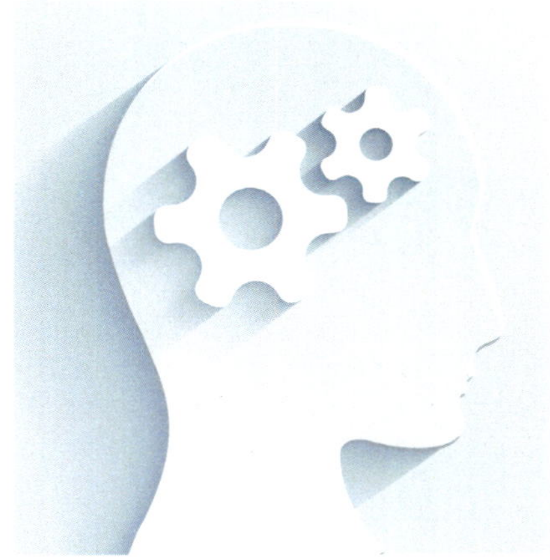

How does fat help maintain our muscle and only for a short time?

Read on: After a long period of glucose (blood sugar) deprivation (like when we diet or when we eliminate carbohydrates), the brain and nerve cells adapt. They can develop the ability to derive half of their energy needs from a special form of fat called a ketone. Ketones can be made from our bodies' fat stores even if we are not consuming fat in our diets. So fat can prevent muscle breakdown to a certain extent. BUT THE BRAIN AND NERVOUS SYSTEM STILL NEED GLUCOSE! Ketones will only go so far. Where will this glucose come from? The body has NO choice but to tap into the only other source of glucose in the body—our protein stores—in other words, our muscle and other lean tissues. Proteins can be broken down by the liver and kidney to be reassembled to look like a molecule of glucose so that the brain doesn't die! This process over time can leave us weak, dehydrate us, create acidity in the blood and compromise our immune system. When half of the body's protein has been used up, we can die. So DO NOT DIET, DO NOT ELIMINATE CARBOHYDRATES OR FAT FROM YOUR DIET EVER! It's all about balance.

Fat makes foods taste delicious and helps you feel satified after eating.

Fat in our diet

General recommendations for fat intake in the dancer's diet range from 20%–30% of total calories. The energy obtained from fat plays an important role for dancers and is used for both high-intensity work and to improve your endurance. One gram of fat supplies 9 calories. One gram of carbohydrate or protein supplies 4 calories. So as you can see, fat supplies lots of calories for energy. But fats also can either improve our health or promote inflammation and heart disease! That is why we want to include foods that contain essential fats and healthy fats (omega-3, polyunsaturated and monounsaturated fats) and reduce not-so-healthy fats (animal or saturated fats, trans fats) to modest amounts.

Type of Fat	Sources
Saturated Fat - Choose less often.	Primarily all animal proteins like red meat, to a lesser extent fish and poultry, full-fat dairy foods, butter, margarine, mayonnaise, shortening, egg yolks
Polyunsaturated Fat - Omega 6 fat contains linoleic acid, an essential fat. Choose more often.	Primarily oils that are liquid at room temperature, like sunflower, safflower, corn, sesame oils
Monounsaturated Fat - Choose more often.	Primarily olive oil, canola oil, avocado, nuts, olives
Omega-3 Fat - An essential fat. Choose more often.	Fish, dark leafy greens, walnuts, flaxseeds and flaxseed oil, chia seeds
Trans Fats - Choose less often.	Hydrogenated and partially hydrogenated oils in prepared foods
Cholesterol - Choose less often.	Cholesterol is found in any food of animal origin like red meat, poultry and to a lesser extent some fish, egg yolks, and full-fat dairy foods. Upper limit for intake per day: 300 mg. Our liver can also make cholesterol, which is needed for cell integrity.

A healthy dance diet reduces saturated fat, trans fats, and cholesterol and includes more monounsaturated fat and omega-3 fat. In practical terms,

THIS IS WHAT YOU SHOULD DO:

1. Choose lean red meat like roast beef or steak if you do eat meat, white meat poultry (no skin)

2. Low-fat or nonfat dairy foods

3. Consume four or five egg yolks per week (unlimited egg whites as they are pure protein and no fat)

4. Reduce butter and mayo and cook with canola oil and/or olive oil and use these as well as flaxseed oil for salad dressings

5. Include nuts in your diet daily and choose fish often

6. Load up on dark leafy greens such as swiss chard, kale, and collard greens

7. Try sliced avocado in your salads and sandwiches for a delicious source of healthy fat

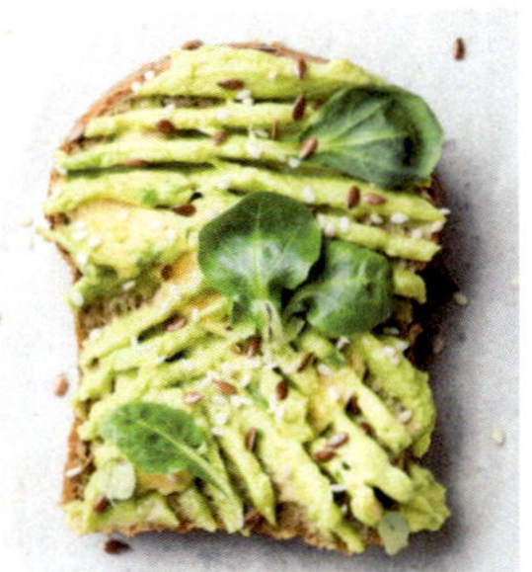
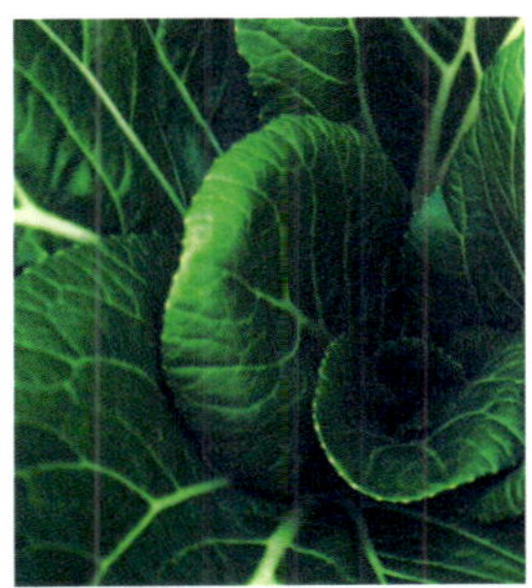
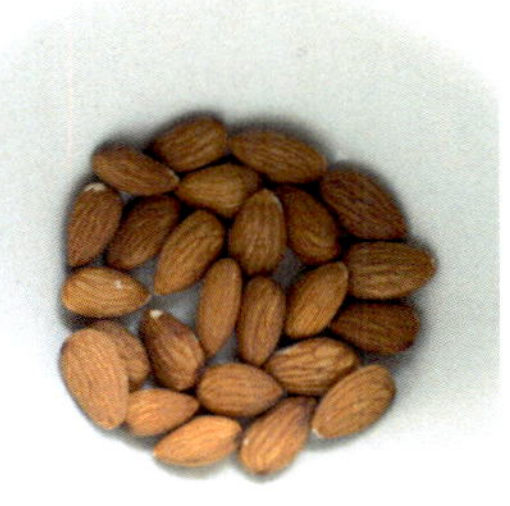

One gram of carbohydrate or protein supplies 4 calories.

If you choose the above foods and keep portions appropriate (see your menu plans and your calorie ranges and suggested servings), that means that you should keep your "added" fat, or the fat that you use for cooking and/or salad dressings to a couple of tablespoons per day, you will be automatically consuming the appropriate amount of fat.

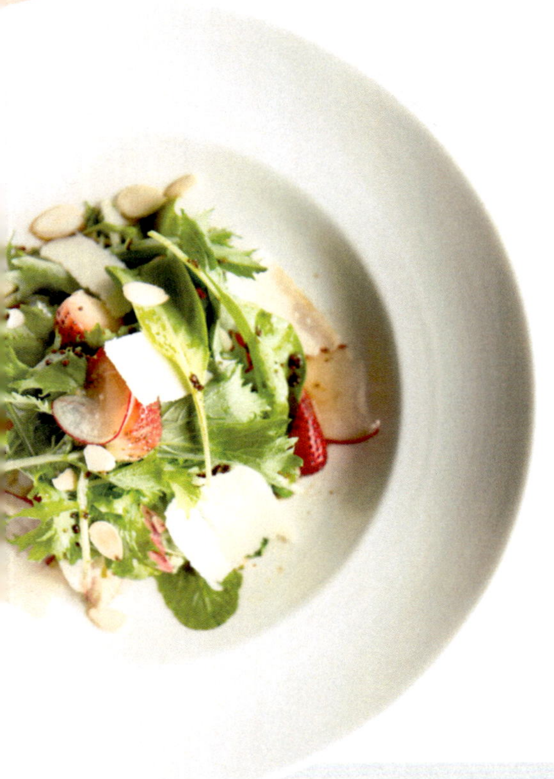

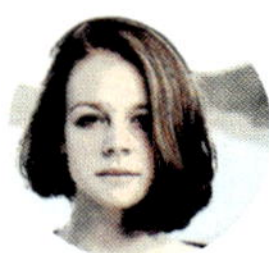

Callie will never eat a dry salad again! She now includes olive oil as part of her salad dressings and knows her mom cooks with olive oil. She has much more energy when she adds some good fat to her meal and notices she is much less hungry in between meals. Food tastes so good when it has some fat included. She also knows that she can have a pat of butter on her homemade muffin at breakfast from time to time and not worry about it. It is about balance and a varied diet!

Taking It to the Next Level:

See the appendix to calculate grams of fat needed per day

Here is another chart for a quick glance at how much fat you should consume on a daily basis for a healthy dance diet. Use the information primarily when you are looking at food labels but don't obsess about having your intake "perfect." Again, if you use your serving size chart or a sample menu in the appendix, you will automatically be consuming an appropriate amount of fat for health. When in doubt, ball park your estimate. Healthy athletic diets contain on average about 25% of their calories from fat give or take a bit.

Grams of fat in your diet

Calorie Intake Per Day	20% Fat	25% Fat	30% Fat
1,600	35.5	44.5	53
1,800	40	50	60
2,100	47	58	70
2,400	55	65	80
2,600	60	70	85
3,000	67	83	100

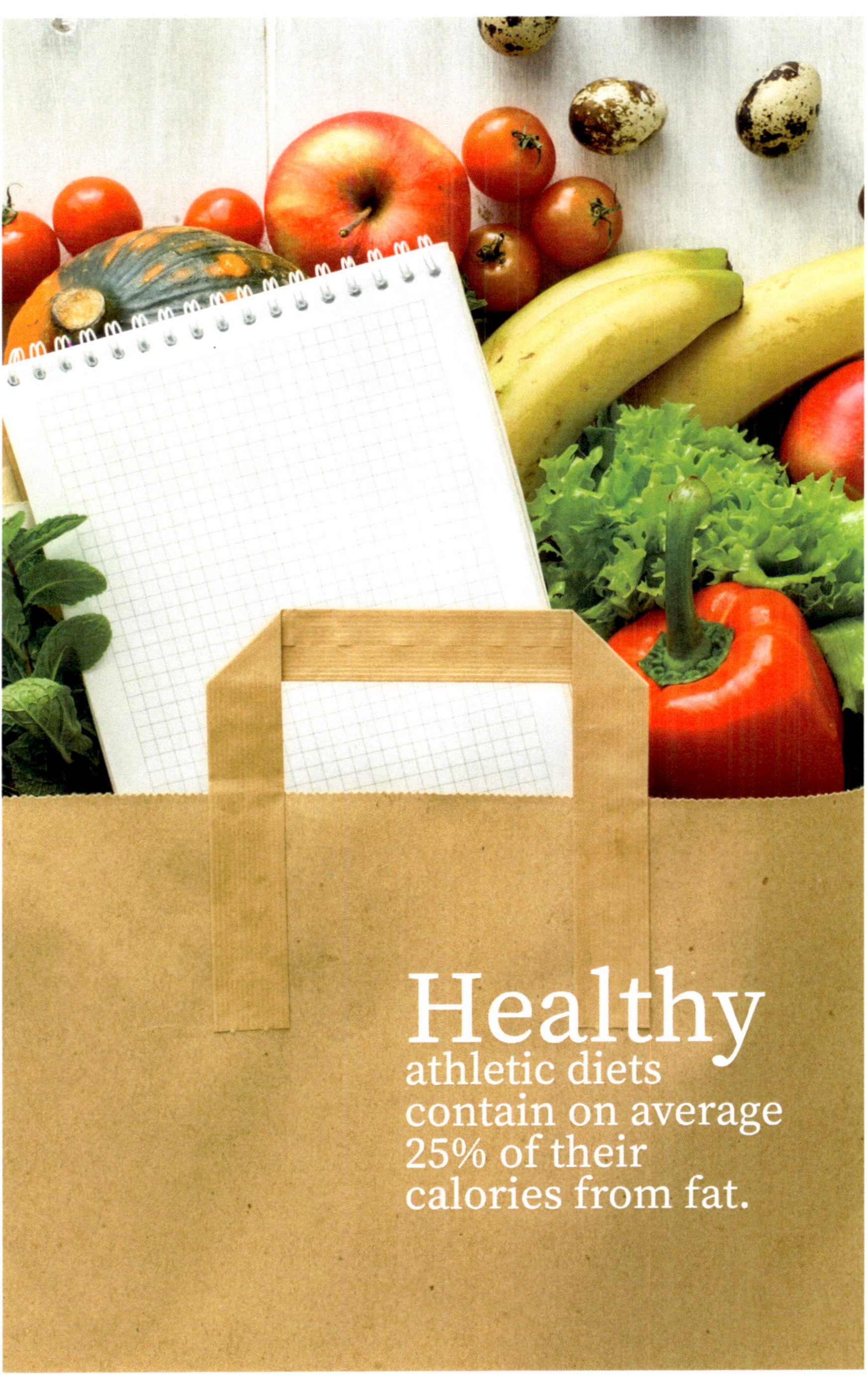
Healthy
athletic diets
contain on average
25% of their
calories from fat.

Review: Chapter 4

1.

Fat helps to keep us lean by preventing overeating and providing energy to dance and exercise. It also makes our food taste good!

2.

Fat can also be used for fuel to spare muscle breakdown if someone "diets" or doesn't consume enough calories/carbohydrates. However, this is not a healthy way to live, and starvation diets are never appropriate.

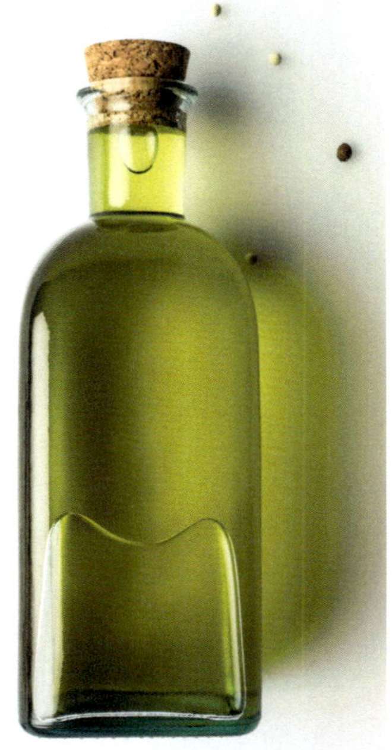

3.

Healthy fats like omega-3 fats (fish and dark leafy greens), monounsaturated fats (olive oil, canola oil, avocado and nuts), and other essential fats like those you get from flax oil or chia seeds can reduce inflammation, be heart healthy and keep cholesterol low.

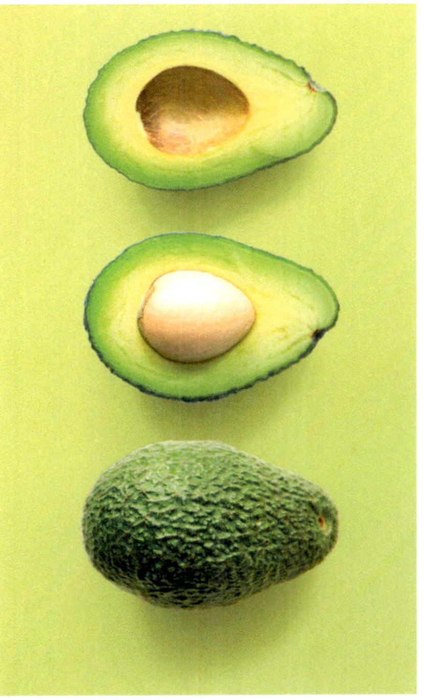

4.

Dietary fat also helps us absorb nutrients in other foods like our fat-soluble vitamins, A, D, E, and K as well as antioxidants.

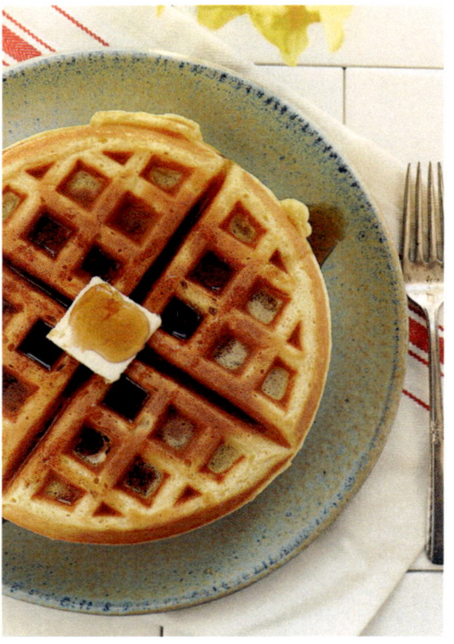

7.

Choose lean red meats (if you eat meat) like roast beef or steak, or cut any visible fat away from a chop or any other meat or poultry.

8.

All foods can fit! If you love butter on your pancakes, please have it! Our diets cannot ever be "perfect," and it is a waste of time living in a "food prison." Just go for variety in all your choices!

5.

There will be a normal amount of fat coming from foods that contain protein like meat or fish or nuts. Keep your added fat like what is used as a salad dressing or for cooking to a couple of tablespoons per day, and you will automatically be consuming adequate fat from your diet.

6.

Reduce saturated fats like those found in fatty meats, skin on chicken, butter, margarine, mayonnaise, shortenings and full-fat dairy foods to reduce inflammation and keep your heart healthy.

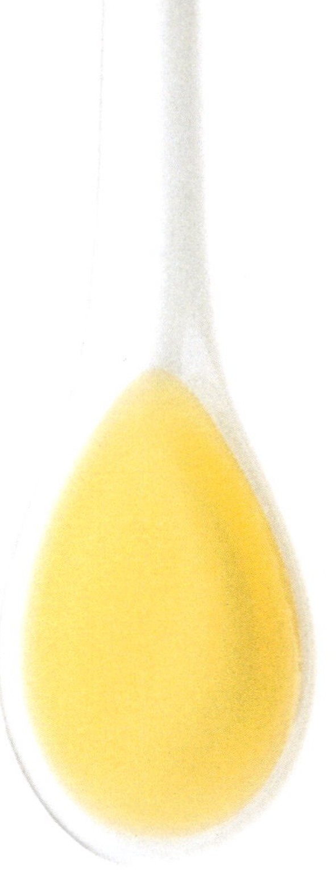

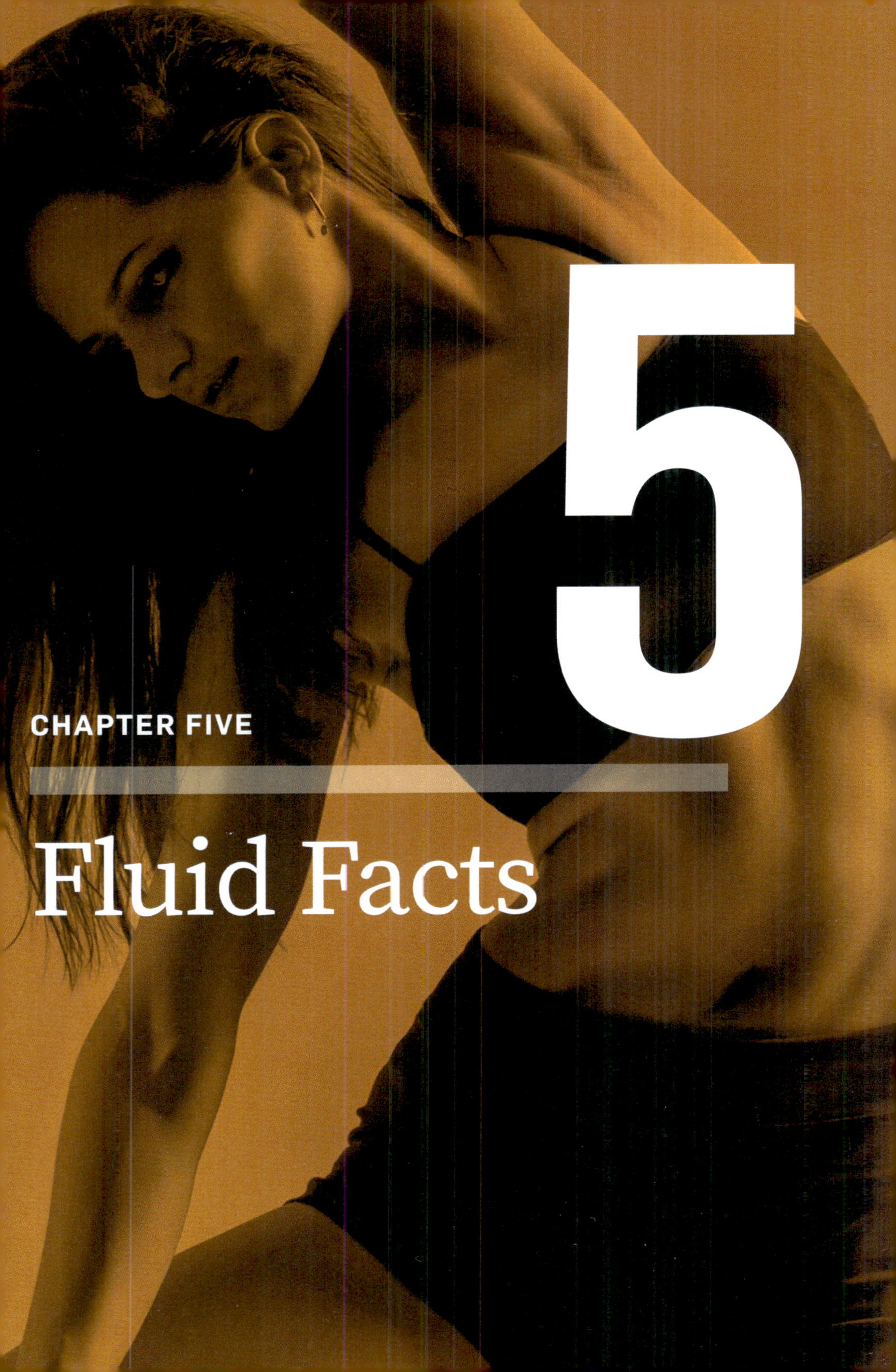

CHAPTER FIVE

Fluid Facts

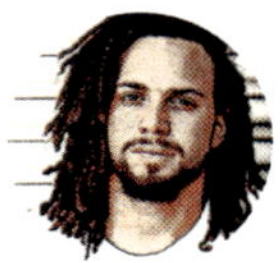

Did You Know?

More than 70% of your lean muscle, blood and brain are water?

According to the American College of Sports Medicine, only you can determine how much water and fluid you need on a daily basis. Fluid needs vary greatly from person to person.

As a dancer, it would help to know that you could possibly lose on average ten to twelve cups of water daily that needs to be replaced to maintain your body's important fluid balance. This depends on your activity level and environment. According to the Mayo Clinic and other leading health organizations, even mild dehydration can lead to loss of energy and constipation.

Dehydration symptoms can include loss of appetite, headaches, dizziness, and lack of mental focus. Not what a dancer wants! There is also evidence to show that drinking enough water can help prevent kidney stones and may be associated with lower risk for colon cancer.

Dehydration is more common than overhydrating, but overhydrating to the point of lowering your blood salt levels is unhealthy and dangerous. Symptoms of overhydration include headache, vomiting, swollen hands and feet, undue fatigue, confusion and wheezing (due to water in the lungs). As a dancer, you want to strike the right balance.

To determine if you are adequately hydrating on a daily basis, simply weigh yourself at the same time each morning before breakfast and after you have emptied your bladder and bowels. Your weight should remain relatively stable and NOT creep downwards.

This weight assumes that you are not trying to lose weight, that you have not eaten salty meals the day before (salt can make you retain water), and you are not retaining water premenstrually. Fluid shifts can make the scale go crazy, so do this as an experiment from time to time. Do not live by the scale.

Another way to determine how much fluid to replace after a long dance or rehearsal day is to weigh yourself in the morning and then weigh yourself after your dance day. For every pound you lose, consume two cups of water to replenish your fluid losses.

Just like the organized dancer that I know you are, don't leave your water intake to chance. Develop a consistent water plan with consumption evenly distributed through your day. Drink often while dancing or exercising. The American Dietetic Association recommends at least two cups of fluids two hours before exertion, followed by another two cups of water approximately fifteen to twenty minutes before endurance exercises. During exercise, replenish fluids every fifteen to twenty minutes, most especially if you are working up a sweat or dancing in a heated environment.

What's best to drink? Shoot for at least five to six cups of water daily to get you close to your goals. Other beverages will contribute the rest. You will get fluids from milk, juices, coffee, and teas. If you take your caffeine in small doses (180 mg/day or the equivalent to an 8-ounce cup of medium strong coffee), it is unlikely that the caffeine will dehydrate you. The good news is that all your fruits and veggies will also provide you with water as well.

Even mild **deyhydration** can lead to the loss of energy and constipation.

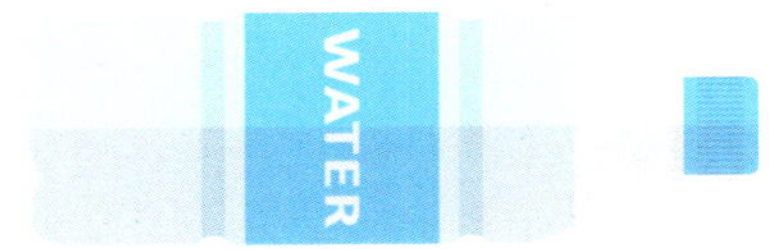

Fast Facts:

Every system of our body needs water every day. And yet most of us do not consume enough water. Water and fluids perform many functions in the dancer's body. Some of these functions include:

1. Serving as a solvent for minerals, vitamins, amino acids, glucose, and many other small molecules.

2. Acting as a lubricant around joints.

3. Serving as a shock absorber inside the eyes, spinal cord, and amniotic sac during pregnancy.

4. Aiding in maintaining the body's optimal temperature.

5. Helping to detoxify the kidneys and liver.

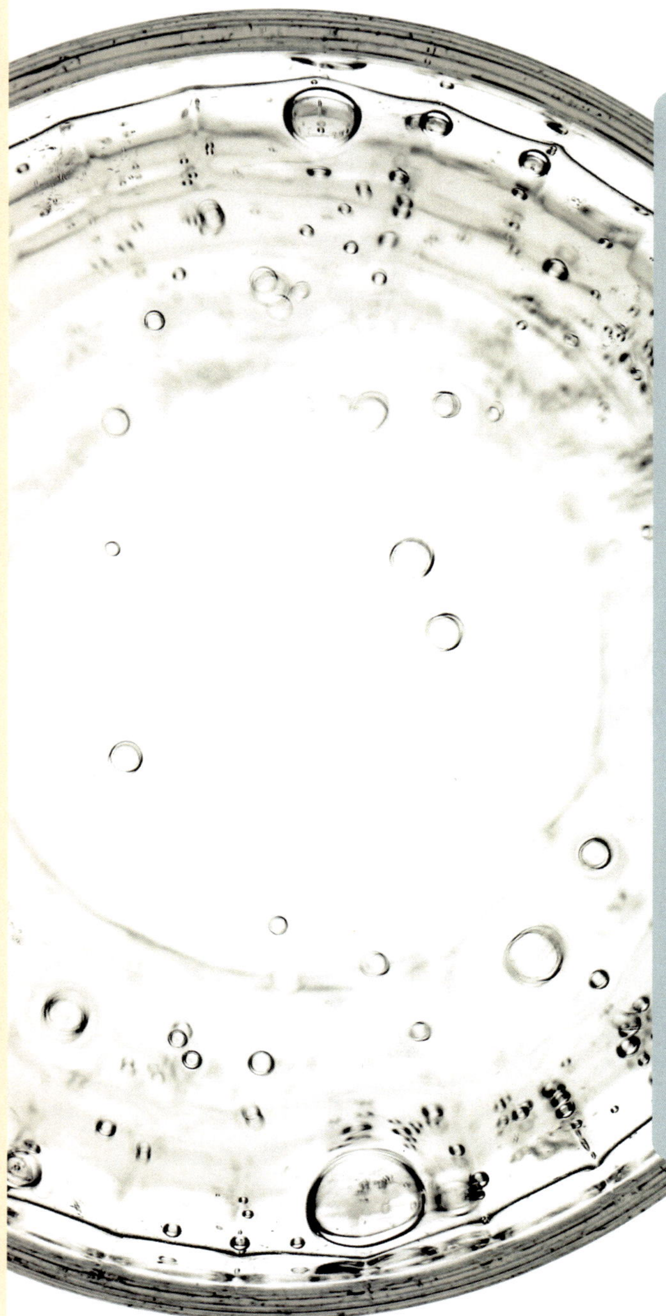

Quick Tip:

Many of my students ask about vitamin water and seltzers for hydration rather than plain water. Is this okay? Vitamin waters DO contain vitamins, and if you are consuming more than one per day, you may be getting too many vitamins in! Use a vitamin water as an occasional treat rather than something you drink every day. Seltzers and other carbonated beverages have not been shown to hurt tooth enamel, so again, have them occasionally as an addition to regular water for your hydration needs.

*

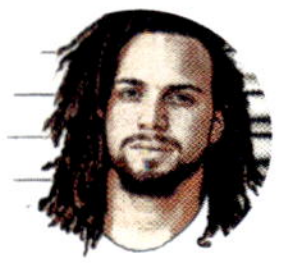

Gregory is going to bring a bottle of water with him to auditions from now on. At home, he will make some iced lightly sweetened peppermint tea and use it to meet his fluid goals. He tries to make up on dance classes on Saturdays, so he will bring a sports replacement drink when he takes two to three classes back to back in a warm studio and sweats a lot. Make a plan and follow it, just like Gregory.

Quick Tip:

We usually hear that we need eight cups a day of water. However, this is not always accurate. As a rule of thumb, one way to calculate your fluid needs is to divide your weight in half. This number in ounces is your recommended daily water intake. So a 160-pound male dancer would need approximately 80 ounces of water, which is about ten cups. (There are 8 ounces in one cup.) If you are the type of dancer who sweats a lot and is extremely active, you might need to add another 20–30 ounces on top of the 80 ounces stated above.

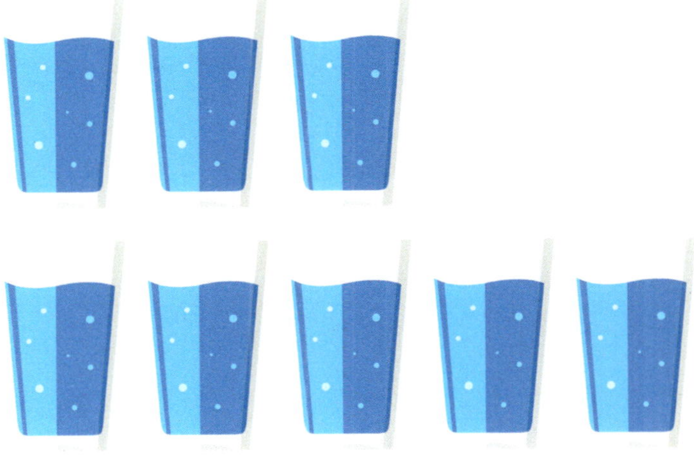

Signs of Dehydration

Early Signs

• Fatigue
• Appetite loss
• Flushed skin
• Heat intolerance
• Light-headedness
• Dark urine with a strong odor

Severe Signs

• Difficulty swallowing
• Stumbling
• Clumsiness
• Shriveled skin
• Sunken eyes and dim vision
• Painful urination
• Numb skin
• Muscle spasms
• Delirium

About Sodium?

If you are participating in an ultra-endurance event or dancing for four hours or more, you should consume a sports drink that contains sodium. Fifty to 120 milligrams consumed during exercise should be sufficient. The sodium content in most sports drinks can range from 8 to 116 milligrams. Check the label. Do not drink sports drinks or any drinks with BVO or brominated vegetable oil. This is an unhealthy ingredient that generally has been eliminated but look at your food labels just to be sure.

Sodium is important because it helps your body absorb fluids and along with sugar, sodium may enhance a drink's taste, which can encourage you to drink more.

The carbohydrates, sodium, and other electrolytes can help your energy and mental focus when dancing in competitions or other situations where you are dancing continuously for more than one hour.

So just like you plan your meals, plan for a healthy fluid intake, and you will have all the energy and mental focus you need to dance well.

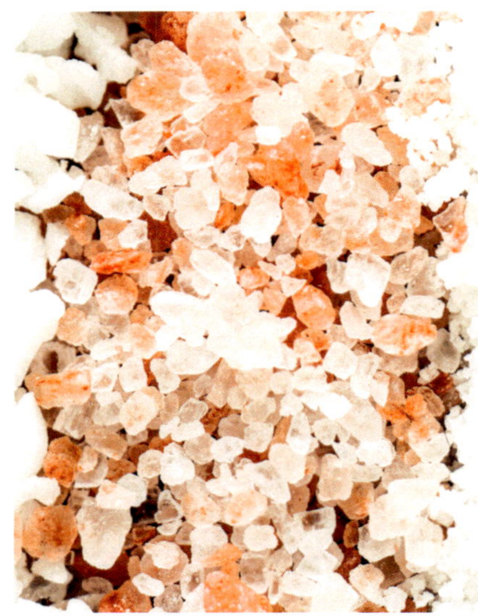

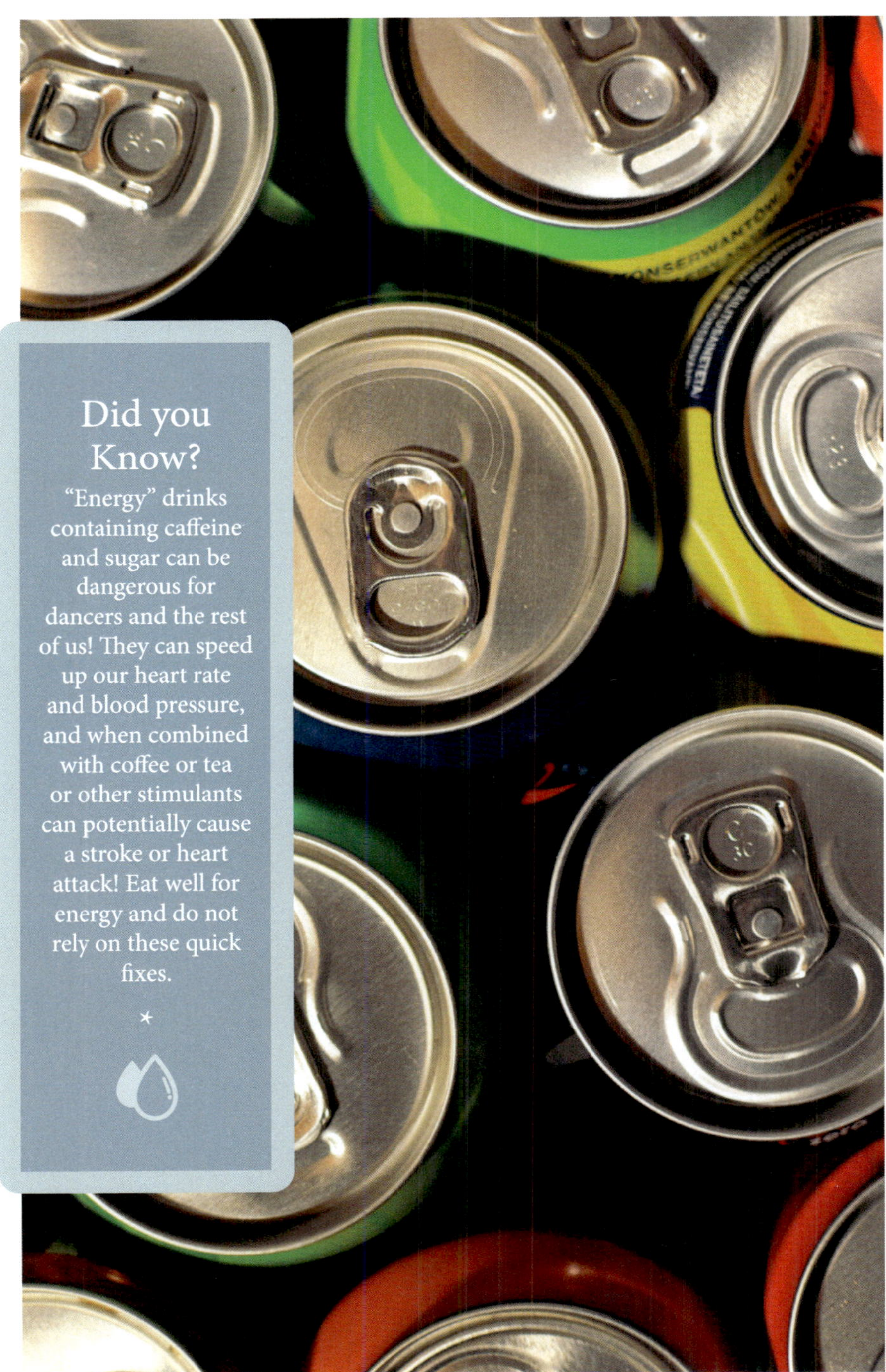

Did you Know?

"Energy" drinks containing caffeine and sugar can be dangerous for dancers and the rest of us! They can speed up our heart rate and blood pressure, and when combined with coffee or tea or other stimulants can potentially cause a stroke or heart attack! Eat well for energy and do not rely on these quick fixes.

*

Review: Chapter 5

1.

Everyone's fluid needs are different.

3.

Make water your fluid of choice. But you also get fluids from milk, juice, coffee and tea, and fruits and veggies.

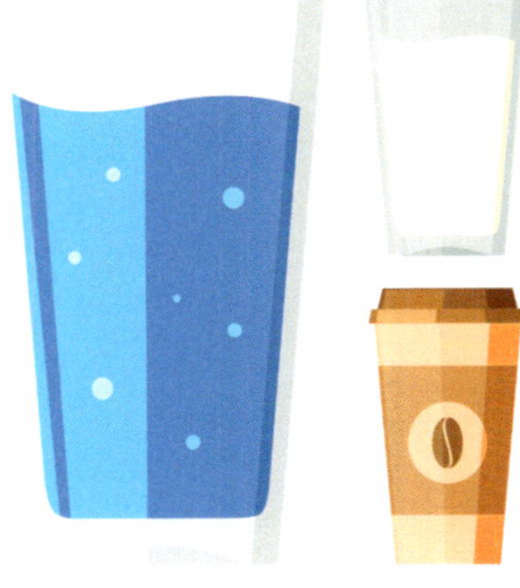

4.

Alcoholic drinks do not provide fluids.

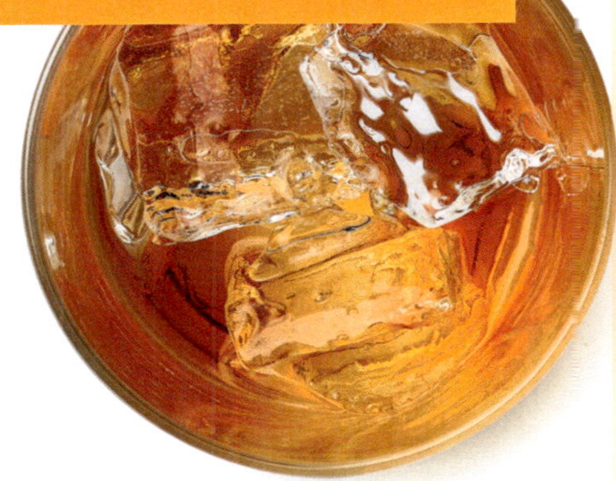

2.

Divide your weight in half. This number could represent the number of ounces of fluids you need on a daily basis.

5.

Sodas often give you too much sugar, so they are not optimal for fluid replacement although an occasional soda or diet soda is okay as a treat.

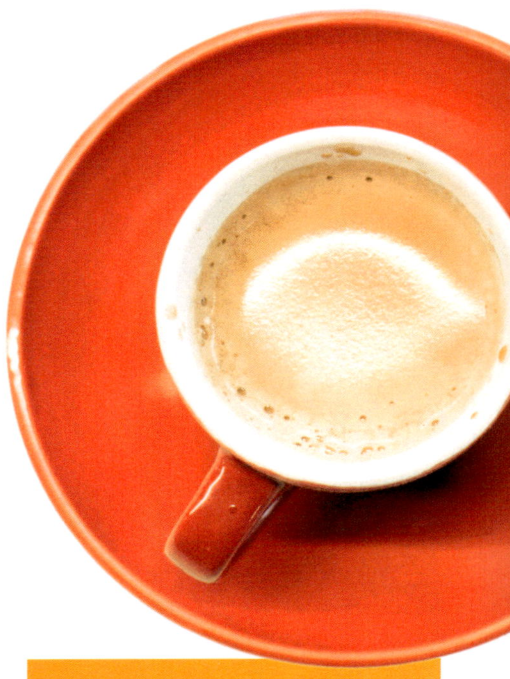

6.

Measure your sweat losses by weighing yourself before a long dance day and after, and replenish two cups of fluids for every pound lost.

8.

Watch out for signs of dehydration. Also be aware of the signs of overhydration.

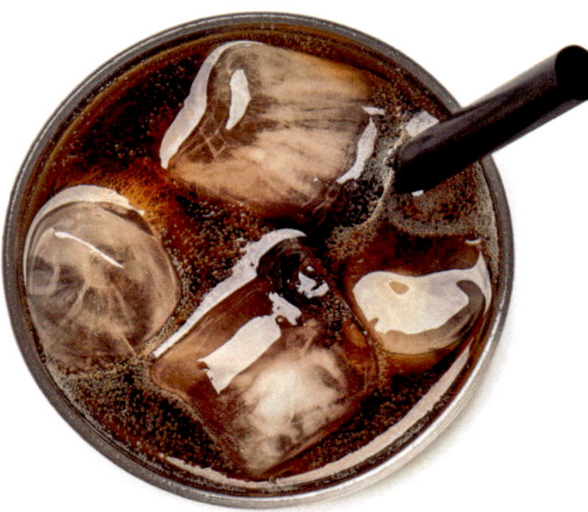

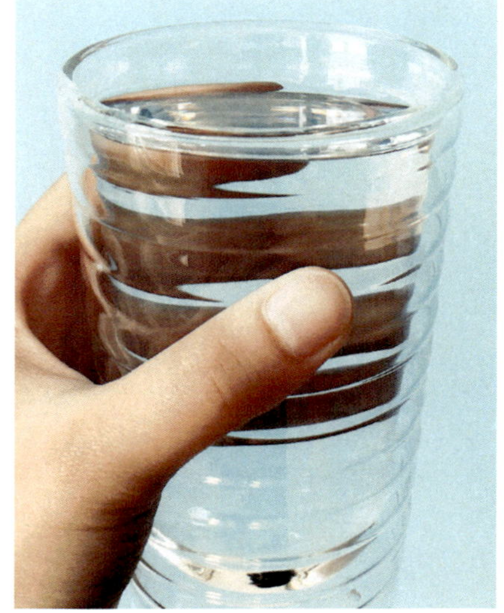

7.

Enjoy a sports beverage like Gatorade if you are dancing and moving continuously for more than an hour.

Too Pooped to Pop? Dancer's Guide to Energy

Where does energy come from?

It is supplied by the food we eat and the liquids we drink. If you feel like you don't have enough energy to make it through your dance day, here are some tips to help remind you of what is important:

1. Get enough sleep. Most dancers need seven to nine hours of sleep each night. See the quick tips box for "sleep hygiene" reminders. Functioning on even one to two hours of sleep less than what you need can affect your energy and concentration.

2. Drink enough water. Take your weight and divide in half. That is the number of ounces of fluids you need daily. Add a couple of extra cups if you sweat a lot. See chapter on fluids. Dehydration can make you extremely tired and can even be dangerous for you as a dancer.

3. Eat enough! Diets that provide 1,600 calories or less do not provide anywhere near the number of calories you need to fuel your dance day. Restrictive eating can leave you feeling tired, mentally unfocused which could lead to injury, and can even cause depression. See chapter on metabolism and take a look at a menu plan for some food ideas to fuel you.

4. Carb up! Carbohydrates are the most important nutrient for energy! They are easily digested and absorbed to keep up your blood sugar and fuel your brain and nervous system. Without them, you will crave sugar and non-nutritious foods that may pick your energy up for a little bit, but then you will crash. See the quick tips box for healthy carbs for energy.

5. Eat some fat! Very low or no-fat diets can impair your energy levels and leave you feeling hungry all the time. A moderate amount of fat is appropriate for dancers. That translates into about 90 grams of fat for male dancers consuming about 2,700 calories per day. That translates into about 70 grams of fat for female dancers consuming about 2,100 calories per day. See quick tips for healthy fats.

6. Eat the right amount of protein. Consuming good-quality protein each time you eat will keep your blood sugar even and prevent hypoglycemia. See quick tips for good protein choices.

7. Watch your iron. Iron deficiency anemia is widespread and a leading cause of fatigue in dancers. Iron levels should be checked by your doctor at your yearly physical. Never supplement with iron unless your doctor tells you to. Good dietary sources of iron include fortified cereals and breads, lean red meat, tofu, kidney beans and spinach. Consuming a vitamin C source with your iron such as orange juice or cooking with lemon juice can increase your absorption of iron.

8. Get all your vitamins and minerals from food first. Don't rely on supplements or let anyone sell you an "energy" supplement. These energy supplements are stimulants that can affect your nervous system and your heart. Stay clear! If you feel like you could benefit from a multivitamin, check out the chapter on vitamins and the appendix for more information.

9. Limit caffeine, alcohol, and sugar. Limit pure sugar intake to 5% of your total calories. (Not the natural sugar you get from carbs, but the refined, white flour sweet stuff like cookies and cakes.) Limit caffeine intake to two eight-ounce cups per day. If you don't drink, don't start; but if you do drink alcohol, limit alcoholic drinks to fewer than three drinks per week.

After reading this chapter, Gregory is making a vow to get more sleep by practicing the tools included in this chapter, and Callie realizes that she needs to pack more snacks for her dance day during the intensive. She will use the snack ideas in this chapter and pack her dance bag with them plus extra water.

Quick Tip:

Sleep Hygiene – Suggestions for Getting Enough Sleep

1. Try to go to bed at the same time each night and wake up at the same time each day even on the weekend.

2. Decompress and unplug. Don't speak on the phone, answer text messages, surf the net or e-mail for at least an hour before sleep. Put your phone away on mute and focus on sleep.

3. Keep your room at a comfortably cool temperature.

4. Relax, don't worry. Create a specific "worry time" during the day when you can worry all you want; when that time is done, you are done "worrying."

5. Watch caffeine and sugar intake late in the day.

6. Create a bedtime routine like warm bath, meditation, reading, journaling, stretching, so that you can wind down.

Quick Tip:

Carbs to Maximize During Your Dance Day:

1. Whole grains such as brown rice, millet, quinoa, buckwheat, oats

2. Whole-grain breads and pastas, cereals and crackers

3. Sweet potatoes and regular white potatoes with skin

4. Whole fruits

5. Whole veggies

6. High fiber choices have 3 or more grams of fiber per serving

Carbs to Minimize:

1. Refined carbohydrates such as cookies, cakes, pies, doughnuts, candy

2. Table sugar, sugary drinks, high-fructose corn syrup

3. White flour breads, pastas and cereals

Quick Tip:

Fats to Maximize

1. Olive oil, canola oil

2. Avocado, nuts, olives

3. Flaxseed oil for salads

4. Omega-3 fats from fish, walnuts, and dark leafy greens

Fats to Minimize:

1. Animal fats (saturated): butter, margarine, mayonnaise, shortening, visible fat on meats, trans fats

Quick Tip:

Good-Quality Proteins to Maximize:

1. Lean red meat, chicken and turkey, fish, eggs, beans, tofu, nuts, low or nonfat dairy foods

Proteins to Minimize:
1. Fatty meats like bacon, sausage, burgers, visible fat on meats, skin on chicken, full-fat dairy

Bonus Snack Ideas

Notice the Combo of Protein and Carbohydrate :

1. Thermos filled with yogurt and fruit smoothie

2. Peanut butter and banana sandwich

3. Three cups air-popped popcorn and glass of skim or almond milk

4. Low-fat Greek yogurt and ½ cup berries

5. One to two slices of turkey breast wrapped around an avocado slice and dipped in salsa

6. 2 tbsp. hummus and whole-grain pita chips

7. Handful of raisins and nuts and ½ cup fresh-squeezed orange juice

8. One cup oatmeal and cup of skim milk or Greek yogurt

9. Hard-boiled egg, whole-grain crackers and handful of baby carrots

10. String cheese, apple and skim milk

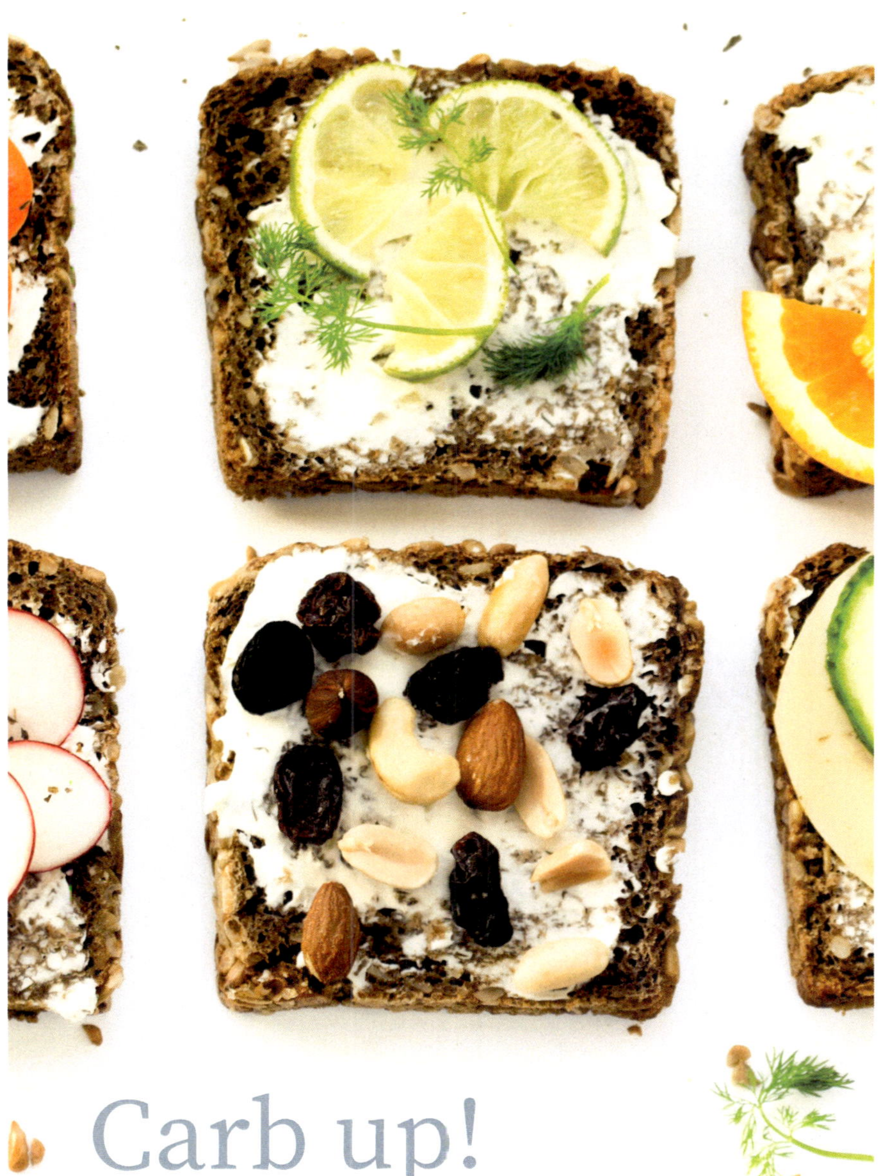

Carb up!
Carbohydroates are the most important nutrient for energy.

Review: Chapter 6

1.

Eat enough. Don't "diet."

2.

Always include a little bit of everything on your plate: carbohydrates, protein, and fat.

3.

Make sure you hydrate.

4.

Get enough sleep.

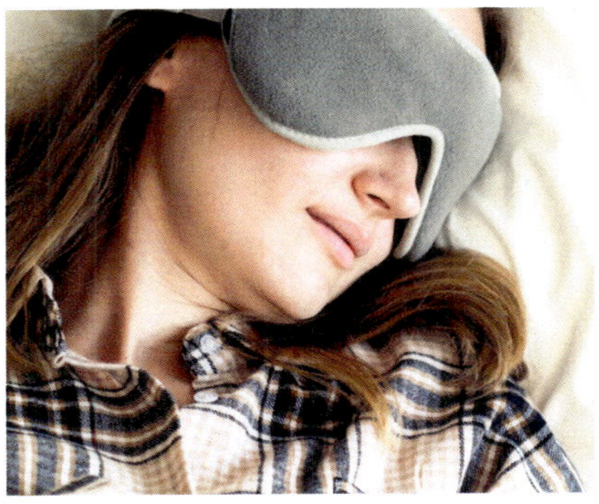

5.

Destress. See the appendix on "Creating a Sacred Space."

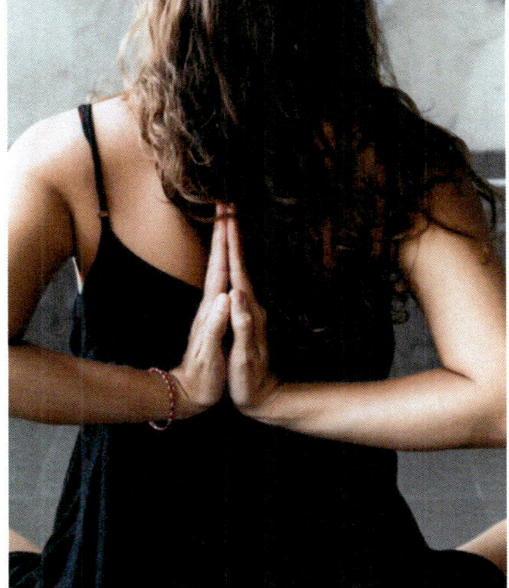

6.

Always have breakfast.

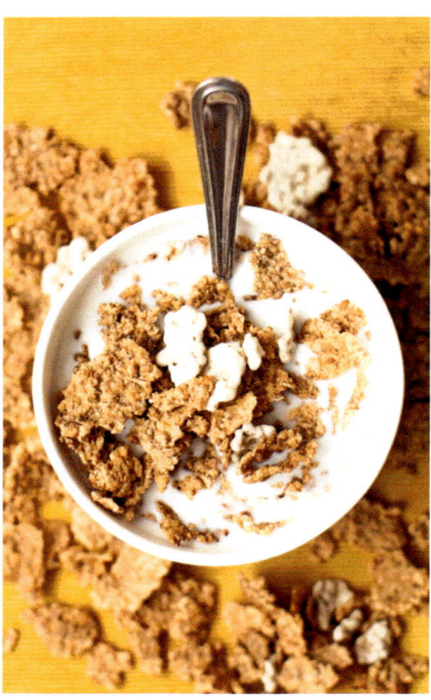

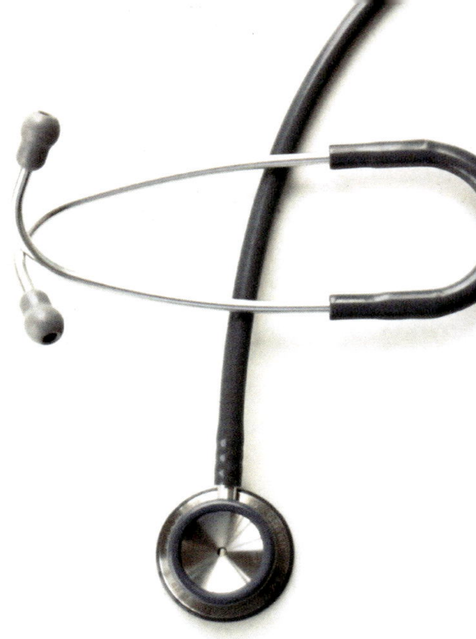

7.

Don't go more than four to five hours without a meal or snack.

8.

Plan healthy snacks to power you through back-to-back classes or rehearsals.

9.

Get a yearly checkup with your doctor to make sure you are not iron deficient.

10.

You can shore up a weak diet with a multivitamin, but supplements themselves will not give you energy. Your lifestyle choices give you energy.

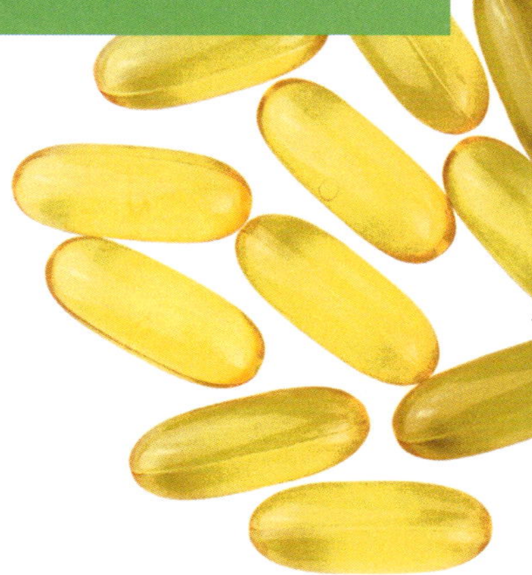

7

Guilt-Free Restaurant Eating

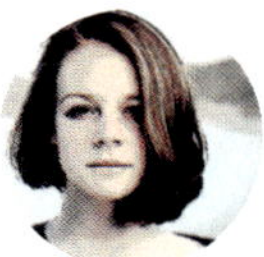

Can busy dancers eat out and still be healthy? Of course you can! You just need to choose wisely and follow the MyPlate recommendations for portions. See the appendix for a version of the MyPlate guidelines.

Most restaurant meals will give you gigantic portions of starch and protein. You will have to look for vegetables or order a side of veggies or fruit to round things out.

Restaurant meals will also give you hefty servings of not-so-healthy fats, sodium, and sugar. How can you manage portions and learn to ask for what you need as a dancer? Here are some simple guidelines that will help you make healthy restaurant choices:

Start each day with a healthy breakfast. Don't starve all day, so you can go haywire at your restaurant dinner. Research shows that those who consume a breakfast that includes whole grains, fruit, and low-fat dairy foods like milk or yogurt generally consume less fat and fewer calories throughout the day.

Balance your food budget. Eat sensibly during the day even if you want to splurge a little at your restaurant dinner.

Start each meal with a big glass of water. Water fills you up without added calories.

Start meals with a fruit or vegetable. In addition to a glass of water, if you are starving when you arrive at the restaurant, order a vegetable-based soup or salad or fruit bowl to nibble on to take the edge off your hunger. These fiber-filled options will fill you up and leave less room for higher calorie foods.

Plan ahead as best you can. Choose restaurants that offer you healthy options like salads, grilled fish and meat, and less fried food. You can also call ahead and ask them to prepare something special that is healthier than what is on the menu. For example, if you love fish and the restaurant usually fries its fish offering, you can call and ask if the fish can be baked or grilled (healthier preparation methods that contain fewer fat calories).

Before ordering, ask lots of questions, such as "how is this prepared?" or "can this be grilled instead of fried?" or "can this be made with olive oil instead of butter?" You get the idea.

Order the smallest size. This goes for fast food restaurants which typically "supersize" their offerings. Even if a larger size seems a good value, decide if you really need the extra calories in the extra portions.

Restaurant portions are HUGE! Typically, you will be served two to three times the portions of carbohydrates and protein that you would make for yourself at home. Ways to control portions are to take half home for lunch the next day, share your meal, or order a few appetizers (they are perfect portions) to make a delicious lunch or dinner.

Order simple dishes. Words on the menu that will hint at healthier cooking methods are grilled, baked, roasted, lightly sautéed, steamed. Descriptives such as creamy, cheesy, deep-fried, tempura, crispy, breaded, or stuffed tell you your meal will be high in calories and high in fat.

Eat sensibly during the day even if you want to splurge a little at your restaurant dinner.

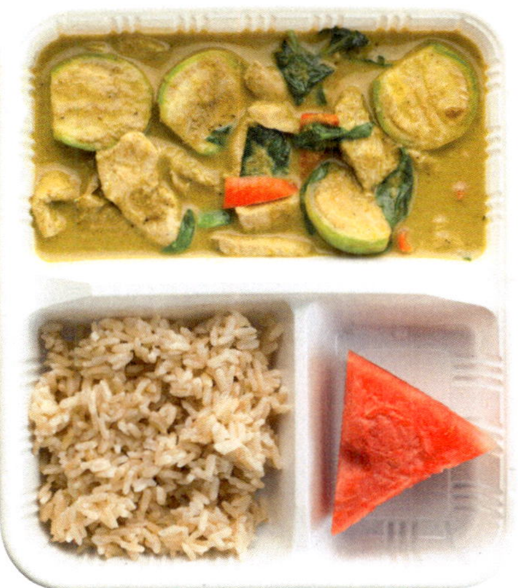

Ask for dressings and sauces "on the side." Salad dressings for example can add hundreds of calories and be double or triple the amount that you would normally use at home.

DO relish your favorite foods! Even if something is fried or cheesy, if you love it and are treating yourself, then by all means, ENJOY it.

Eat slowly and savor every bite. Eating too quickly and not paying attention to what you eat is a sure way to overeat! It takes twenty minutes or so for the nerves in the stomach to signal the brain that you are full. So if you eat your fettucine alfredo in ten minutes by wolfing it down, you will still feel hungry if you do not wait another ten or fifteen minutes to let everything settle. So if you order another serving and eat it, you will be absolutely STUFFED and uncomfortable a half hour after you eat. Take your time and allow your body's signals of fullness and hunger to work for you.

Stop eating when you are full!
Just because you spent $30 on your chicken and pasta doesn't mean that you have to be a member of the "clean plate club"! If you take your time eating and allow twenty to thirty minutes after you eat to feel your fullness, then you can ask the waitperson to bag up what is left and take it home. Do not overstuff yourself just because you spent a lot of money on your meal and feel like you should finish it no matter what. You will feel guilty and miserable after your restaurant meal if you eat to the point of being so full you have to unbuckle your belt buckle. Take care of YOU by paying attention to how you feel. Focus on the conversation and companionship of family and friends rather than on overdoing food.

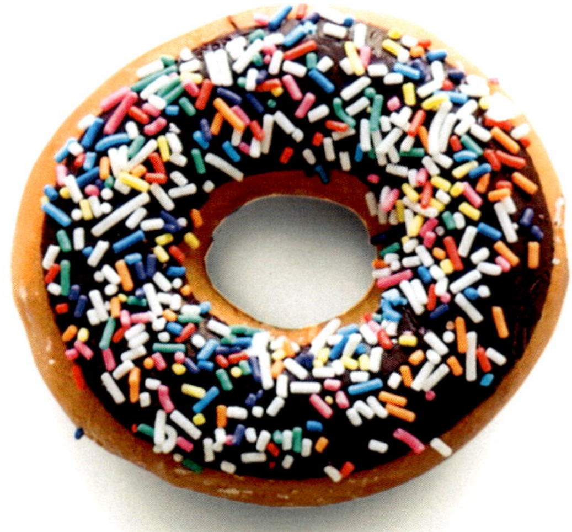

Sugar intake should be 10% or less of your total calorie intake for a day.

Going out to eat doesn't have to mean that you throw your health out the window. Plan ahead as best you can, make healthy choices, eat slowly and enjoy and stop eating when you are full.

Desserts are okay for dancers!
Sometimes, you only need a little bite of something sweet to feel satisfied. Sharing desserts can be fun and delicious. A once in a while treat is perfectly healthy and acceptable. Remember that the recommendation for sugar intake is to be 10% or less our total calorie intake for the day. Eat accordingly.

Alcohol contains 7 calories per gram and is processed as fat by our livers. I do not recommend alcohol on a regular basis for dancers. What is considered "one" drink? That would be 5 oz. of wine, 1.5 oz. of hard liquor or a 12-ounce beer. One or two alcoholic drinks per week can be considered within healthy limits for dancers. A cautionary tale: alcohol is addictive, toxic to the liver, can elevate risk for breast cancer, makes you excrete calcium and adds extra calories that a dancer might not need. Be sensible and exercise control in this area. If you don't drink, don't start.

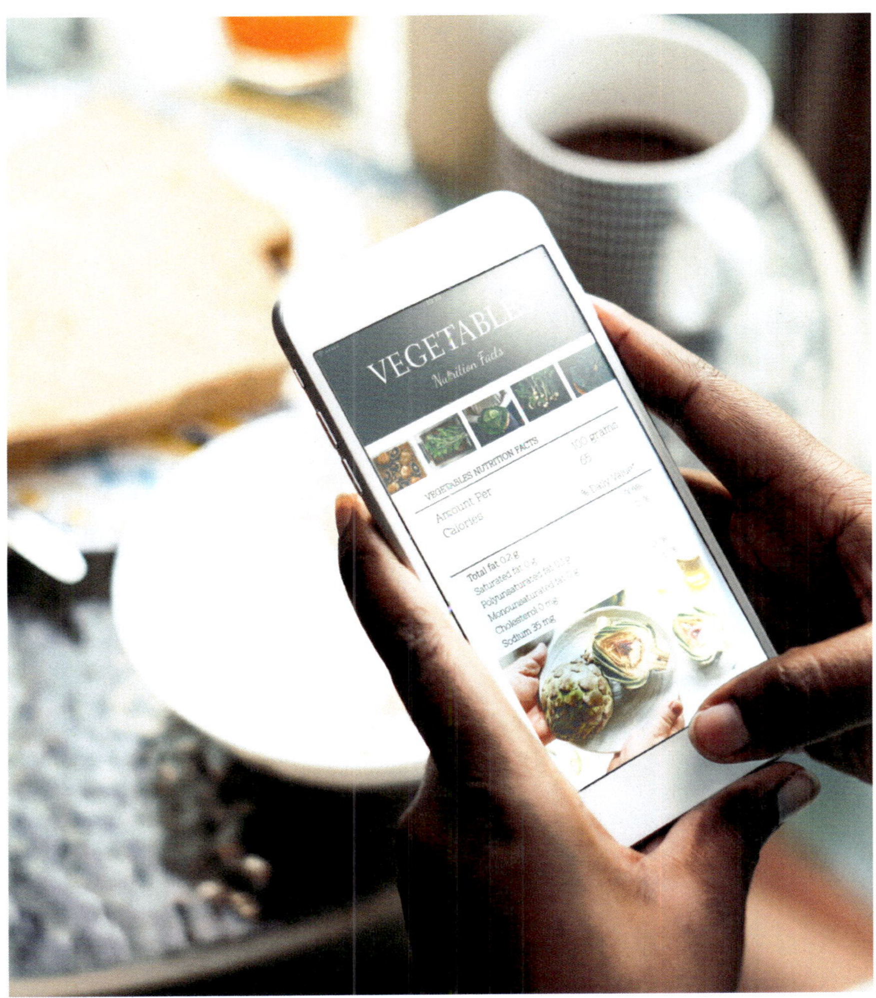

Callie is going to explore restaurant menus online before she and her friends try them. Then she will be prepared. She and her roommates have decided on sharing dishes and bringing some food home for lunches the next day. Callie feels comfy ordering her favorite pasta dish knowing that it is okay to include your favorites and enjoy her meal without guilt! It is all about balance!

Review: Chapter 7

1.

All foods can fit into a dancer's diet. You don't have to be perfect all the time. Choose your favorite foods when you eat out and just watch portions.

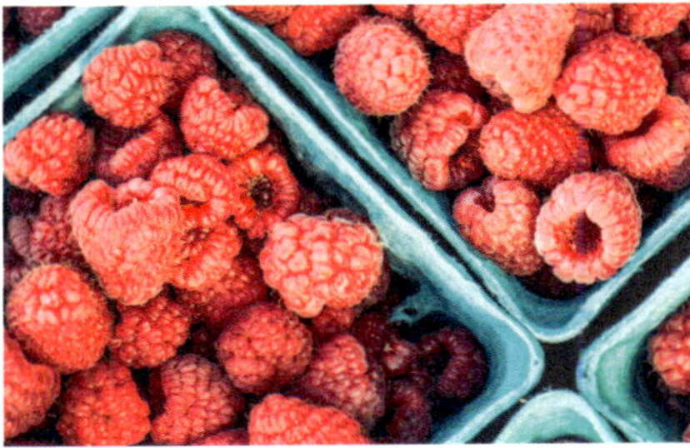

2.

Eat slowly and enjoy and savor each bite. By slowing down, you can recognize when you are physically full (feeling comfortable and not stuffed).

3.

Remember that it takes twenty to thirty minutes after you eat for the nerves in the stomach to send a message to the brain that you are full. If you wolf your food down in ten minutes and decide you need a second dinner, in about half an hour, you will be so stuffed that you will be miserable and wonder WHY you ate so much.

4.

Focus on good conversation and good company rather than huge portions of unhealthy food at restaurants.

5.

Google the menu ahead of time so that you know if there will be healthy choices available for you, especially if you have food allergies or follow a specific diet for health reasons, such as being gluten-free. You can call the chef ahead of time and make your special food requests. Restaurants are happy to oblige you, especially if you are courteous enough to call ahead."

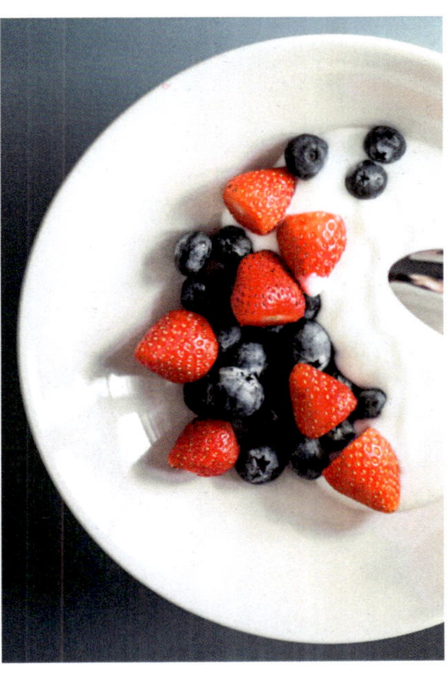

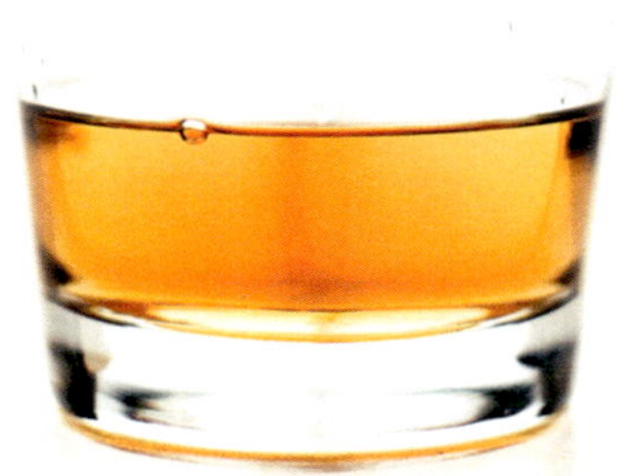

8.
Round out the large portions of protein and starch with a side salad, soup or veggie.

9.
Fruit for dessert is a great option.

6.
Watch alcohol intake. Keep alcoholic drinks to a minimum if you do drink. If you don't drink, don't start.

7.
Choose restaurants that give you healthy options.

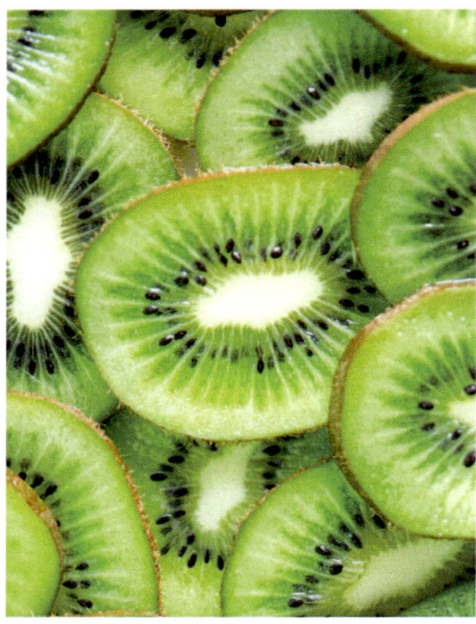

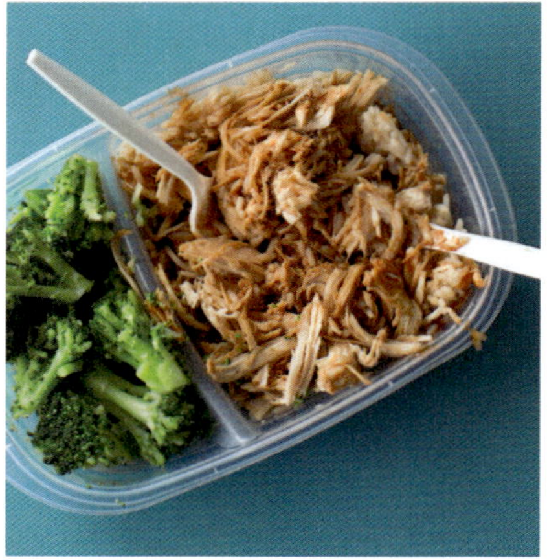

10.
Ask for what you want: a healthier cooking method, less sodium, less fat, dressings and sauces on the side, a fruit or veggie side, sparkling water to drink, etc.

Food Shopping Heathfully

Do you get confused when shopping for food? Do you know what "hot spots" to look for on the food label that would tell you if your food is healthy? These are questions this chapter will cover and more. Of course, I know dancers are busy, but your health is in your hands when it comes to your nutrition. With just some simple guidelines, you will be able to choose healthful foods which can be prepared easily, especially if you don't have time!

So far, you have learned about the three macronutrients essential for dancers and even us regular folks: carbohydrates, proteins, and fats. All of these foods provide calories for energy, fiber to keep you feeling satisfied and for gut health, and vitamins and minerals for healthy bones, skin, teeth, heart and immunity which your dancing body and mind need every day, 24/7.

We now have to put that knowledge into practice by choosing healthy foods that will provide us with the building blocks for energy and health. Let's talk first about purchasing your food and the guidelines for shopping healthfully.

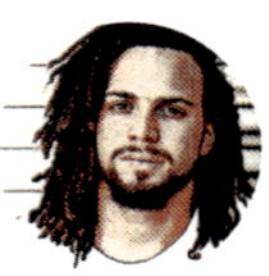

Before moving to New York, Gregory lived with his mom and dad and never did food shopping on his own. He finds it a bit confusing and label reading is not easy. The government has designed a new food label that manufacturers will be required to use by 2018. The serving size will be larger and based on a more realistic portion. But for now, he would like some simple information to help him choose healthful foods.

1. Make a list:

Before you head to the supermarket, health food store, or corner neighborhood grocery, take the time to make a list. It will save you time and money.

How do I make a list? If you can, write out your meal ideas for a week or at least a few days. List the days you will have time to cook and those days that you won't. Plan for those days that will be too busy to do much food preparation by purchasing convenience items like a rotisserie chicken, a bag of precut salad, perhaps even a frozen meal entrée or frozen veggies. If you know Friday night will be pizza night, shop for salad, milk, and fruit to round out the meal. See sample list at end of chapter.

Here is a sample split pea soup label with some quick and easy guidelines especially made for a dancer's health:

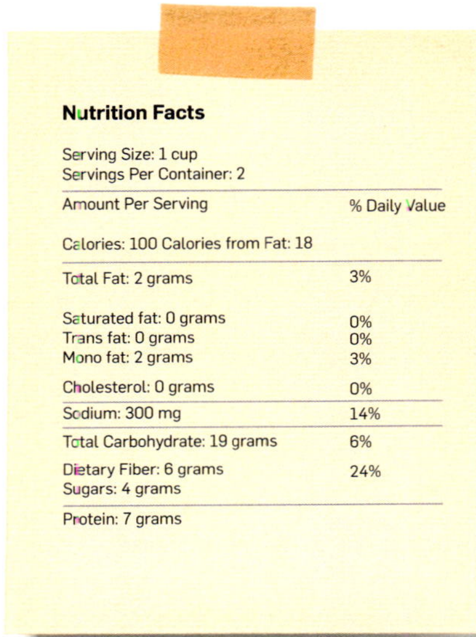

Organize your list. Make sure you are including your basics: cereals, breads, rice, potatoes, pasta, crackers, fruits, veggies, lean meats and poultry, beans, soups, eggs, peanut butter, yogurt, cheese, tuna and other fish.

Beyond the basics. Don't forget your healthy snacks. Stock your pantry with whole-grain pretzels, nuts of all kinds, lightly salted popcorn, low-fat frozen yogurt, and of course, lots of fruit: fresh, canned and dried.

2. Your Strategy:

Don't go shopping when you are hungry. You will be tempted to purchase everything in the store! It is easier to stick to your list when you are not starving, so eat before you go.

Set a routine. If you can establish a day and time that makes it easy for you to shop, it will prevent you from running out of food. It is no fun coming home from a long dance day filled with classes, rehearsals, school, part-time job, etc., only to stare into an empty fridge. Then what??

Save money. Use coupons and ask if your store has a rewards program. Talk to the customer service representative, and they will set you up.

The labels. They are the dancer's best friend. They are your best tool for not wasting money on unhealthful items.

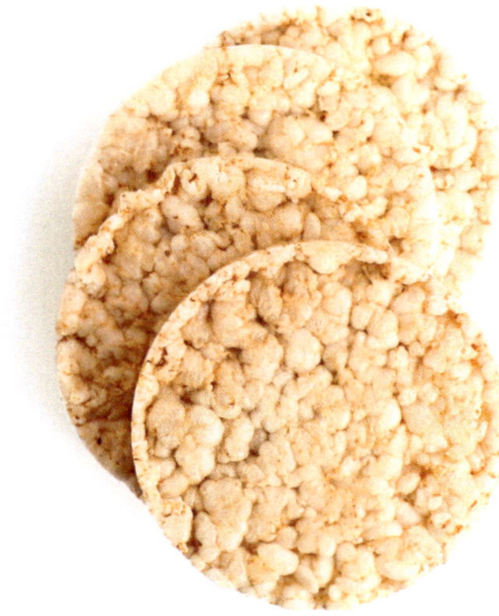

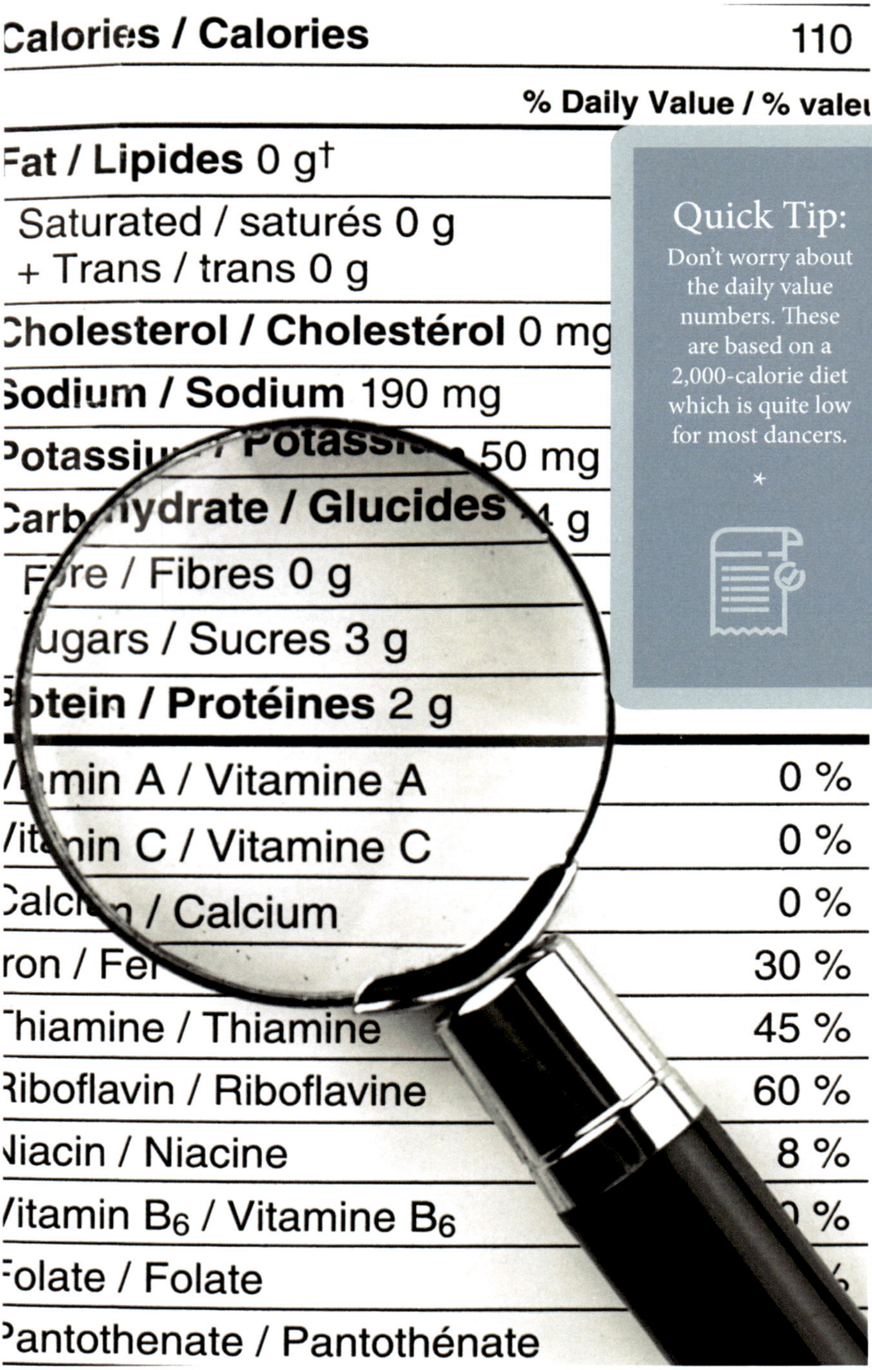

Calories / Calories | 110

% Daily Value / % vale

Fat / **Lipides** 0 g†

 Saturated / saturés 0 g
 + Trans / trans 0 g

Cholesterol / Cholestérol 0 mg

Sodium / Sodium 190 mg

Potassium / Potassium 50 mg

Carbohydrate / Glucides 4 g

 Fibre / Fibres 0 g

 Sugars / Sucres 3 g

Protein / Protéines 2 g

Vitamin A / Vitamine A | 0 %

Vitamin C / Vitamine C | 0 %

Calcium / Calcium | 0 %

Iron / Fer | 30 %

Thiamine / Thiamine | 45 %

Riboflavin / Riboflavine | 60 %

Niacin / Niacine | 8 %

Vitamin B$_6$ / Vitamine B$_6$ | 0 %

Folate / Folate

Pantothenate / Pantothénate

Okay! Let's break down the label and look for "hot spots."

1. Serving size: look at what an actual serving is and know if you eat 2 servings (or the whole can) of soup that you have to double all the numbers on the label.

2. Calories and calories from fat (this will change in 2018 as calories from fat will be eliminated): remember that consuming enough calories throughout your busy dance day is challenging, so don't worry so much about judging how many calories you are consuming. Just get them in. They all add up to good energy. Fat is one of the three important nutrients for health, so we don't want to completely eliminate fat from the diet. We just want to make sure that we keep our hearts healthy by not overconsuming the less healthy fats that are found in some foods.

> ## Hot Spot for Dancers:
> Calories from fat should be 1/3 or less than total calories per serving. This amount has been established in science to be healthful for us as dancers.

3. Total fat: We have learned that the type of fat that we consume is very important. To keep a dancer's cardiovascular systems healthy and to reduce inflammation, look at the type of fat that is in your food:

• **Saturated fats:** This fat comes from our animal foods like red meat, full-fat dairy, egg yolks, and to a lesser extent, poultry and fish. Any fat that is solid at room temperature like butter, margarine, mayonnaise, or shortening acts in our bodies like a saturated fat. These fats can elevate cholesterol and promote inflammation. Reduce their intake in your diet as best you can. No one can ever eliminate saturated fats completely, so just be reasonable in lowering your intake.

• **Trans fats:** These fats are manufactured fats that were once liquid at room temperature and therefore healthier, but because of processing to increase their shelf life, they act in our bodies like saturated fats. Go as low on these fats as possible.

• **Monounsaturated fats and polyunsaturated fats:** These fats come from plants and seeds like sunflowers, corn, sesame and olives. These are the healthiest choices for dancers. Look for the bulk of your fat to come from these healthful liquid oils.

> ## Hot Spot for Dancers:
> Total fat grams should be 3 grams of fat or less
> per 100 calories (in calories per serving).

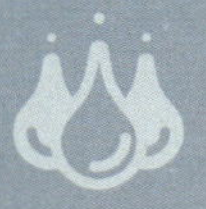

4. Cholesterol: Cholesterol is only present in an animal-based food like meat, poultry, fish, egg yolks and full-fat dairy. Our livers have the ability to help regulate our cholesterol levels, but health guidelines tell us to consume less than 300 mg of cholesterol daily from all sources.

5. Sodium: Excess sodium can elevate blood pressure in some people. More importantly for dancers , however, is the fact that excess sodium increases the excretion of calcium in the urine. For bone health, a healthy dance diet should contain 2,400 mg of sodium or less on a daily basis. If your frozen dinner entrée, for example, contains 1,000 mg of sodium, you may want to look at lower sodium options.

> ## Hot Spot for Dancers:
> Under 200 mg of sodium per serving is
> a good guide.

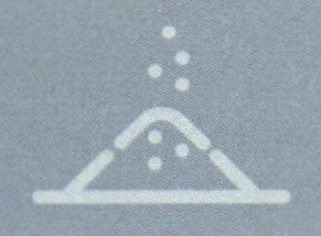

6.Total Carbohydrate: Remember that carbohydrates are the number one fuel source for the dancer. Consuming a low-carbohydrate diet will seriously impair your ability to dance let alone feel good. One serving of carbohydrate = 15 grams of carbohydrate. So in our soup example, one cup of soup gives you one carbohydrate serving (which comes from the carbohydrates in the split peas.) Most dancers need 200–250 grams of carbohydrates every day.

7. Fiber: Fiber is essential for good gut health to eliminate excess cholesterol and to keep up our blood sugar and energy. Foods with a good amount of fiber fill us up and promote satiety. Most dancers need to consume anywhere between 25–35 grams of fiber per day.

Consuming a low-carbohydrate diet will impair your ability to dance let alone feel good.

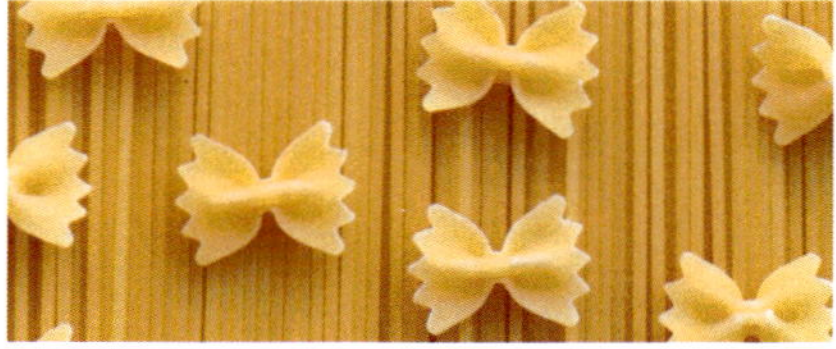

> **Hot Spot for Dancers:**
> Any food that has 3 grams of fiber or more
> per serving is considered a good fiber source.

8. Protein: It is a good idea to get a little protein in every time you eat. Protein balances out your carbohydrates to give you sustained energy and mental focus and to repair muscle. One ounce of protein = 7 grams of protein. In our example, 1 cup of soup is equivalent to one ounce of meat, poultry, or fish. Most female dancers need approximately 80 grams of protein daily; most male dancers need approximately 90–100 grams of protein daily.

9. Ingredients: In addition to looking at the food label, look at the ingredient list! The ingredients in your food are labeled in descending order of volume. That means that the first ingredient listed is in the recipe in the greatest amount and so on down the list. Make sure your first 3 ingredients are real food, not chemicals or additives. And if you see sugar in there, as long as it is close to the last ingredient, you can be assured that it is present in small amounts.

If you see a sugar listing on the label but cannot see sugar as an ingredient, that is because there has been no sugar added. The grams of sugar listed are natural sugars in the food (this will be the case with all carbohydrates, dairy foods, and beans). Natural sugars in carbohydrates are what feed our brains, nervous system and working muscles every moment of every day and are beneficial to consume.

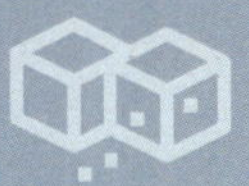

> **Hot Spot for Dancers:**
> 10 grams of sugar or less per serving (if there is
> added sugar in the ingredient list) is a good guide.

If your favorite food has a bit more, have it. Just balance out the rest of your day. NOTE: The new food label in 2018 will have a listing for "added sugars." The fewer "added sugars" the better.

If you see the words hydrogenated or partially hydrogenated, this tells you that there are trans fats in your food. They should be one of the last ingredients if they are present at all.

Using these simple guides and tips will help you get the most from your shopping experience and help you be a savvy shopper. It may take you some time to use all of them but start slowly and practice.

Now that you have gone shopping for healthy food, what are the healthiest ways to prepare your food?

Here is a chart of the best ways to prepare your food to preserve the nutrients that you need to be a healthy dancer:

What It Is And How To Use It

PRESSURE COOKING: A pressure cooker is a pot that has a locking lid. It cooks food quickly and healthfully by creating steam under pressure, which raises the cooking temperature. This method works the best with beans, grains, and vegetables. Watch your cooking time as foods can cook quickly. Also when cooking grains and beans, do not fill the cooker to the top as these foods need room to expand.

STEAMING: This method retains the most nutrients as the food is not placed in water. Almost any food that can be boiled may be steamed, especially vegetables. You can buy a metal or bamboo steamer and a larger pot will allow you to steam more food at one time.

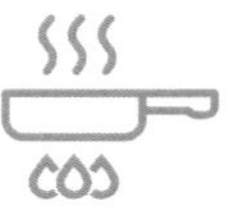

STIR-FRYING: Stir-frying is a fast way of cooking small, uniform-sized pieces of food, most commonly mixed vegetables and strips of beef, chicken, or small pieces of fish. You can stir-fry in a wok or a small frying pan. Stir-frying uses relatively little oil and the temperature is kept high to cook quickly on top of the stove. If desired, you can use broth, wine or nonstick cooking spray instead of oil. This method requires constant stirring and a watchful eye.

BROILING AND GRILLING: These cooking methods expose food to direct heat, leaving it crispy on the outside and flavorful and juicy on the inside. They can be done in a conventional oven or even a good toaster oven. Broiling and grilling work well with meat, poultry, fish, vegetables, and even fruit! You can marinate your food with some flavorful herbs and spices and sauces.

Place your foods about four inches from the heat source and as they cook, baste them with broth, marinade or juice. Turn over when they begin to brown and cook the underside.

ROASTING: Roasting foods like meat or veggies means that they will be cooked slowly in the dry heat of an oven. Roasting temperatures are typically higher than baking temperatures. Almost any kind of meat works well with this method and require a good roasting pan to catch drippings. Get a meat thermometer to make sure your food is cooked to the proper temperature. Vegetables can be roasted on a baking sheet and will brown when ready. Use herbs and garlic and marinades for flavor.

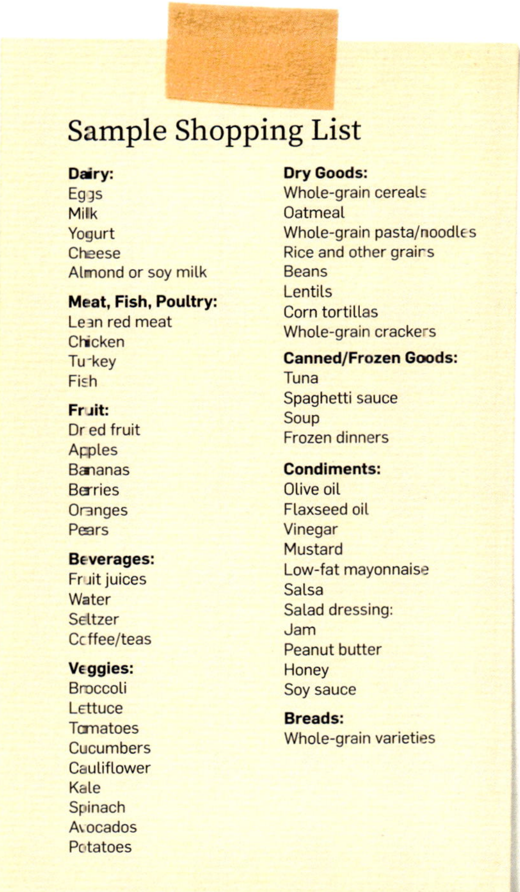

Sample Shopping List

Dairy:
Eggs
Milk
Yogurt
Cheese
Almond or soy milk

Meat, Fish, Poultry:
Lean red meat
Chicken
Turkey
Fish

Fruit:
Dried fruit
Apples
Bananas
Berries
Oranges
Pears

Beverages:
Fruit juices
Water
Seltzer
Coffee/teas

Veggies:
Broccoli
Lettuce
Tomatoes
Cucumbers
Cauliflower
Kale
Spinach
Avocados
Potatoes

Dry Goods:
Whole-grain cereals
Oatmeal
Whole-grain pasta/noodles
Rice and other grains
Beans
Lentils
Corn tortillas
Whole-grain crackers

Canned/Frozen Goods:
Tuna
Spaghetti sauce
Soup
Frozen dinners

Condiments:
Olive oil
Flaxseed oil
Vinegar
Mustard
Low-fat mayonnaise
Salsa
Salad dressing:
Jam
Peanut butter
Honey
Soy sauce

Breads:
Whole-grain varieties

You may find that there are still days when you get caught short and look in the fridge and see nothing. You might resort to a phone app like seamless.com for ordering food, which is absolutely fine. Just know what you are ordering and how it fits into your food plan. See the chapter on restaurant eating for some general tips.

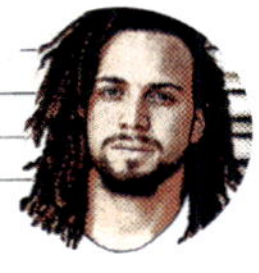

Gregory is going to use a shopping list each week. He will loosely follow the recommended "hot spots" for dancers as a guide. He will focus on more fresh food and check his snack labels for sodium, and saturated and trans fats. You can choose healthfully too.

Review: Chapter 8

1.

Make a list and follow it.

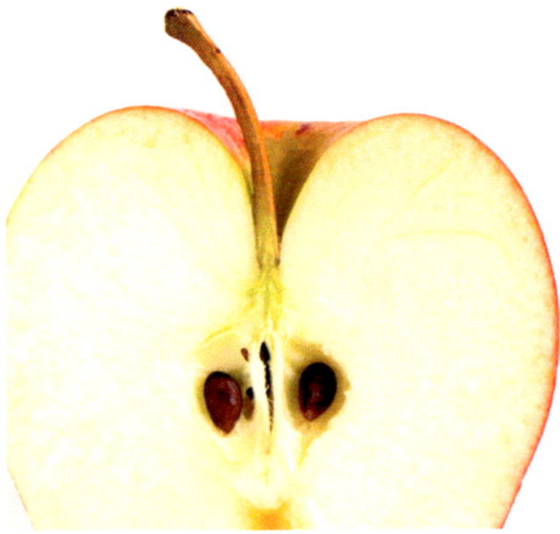

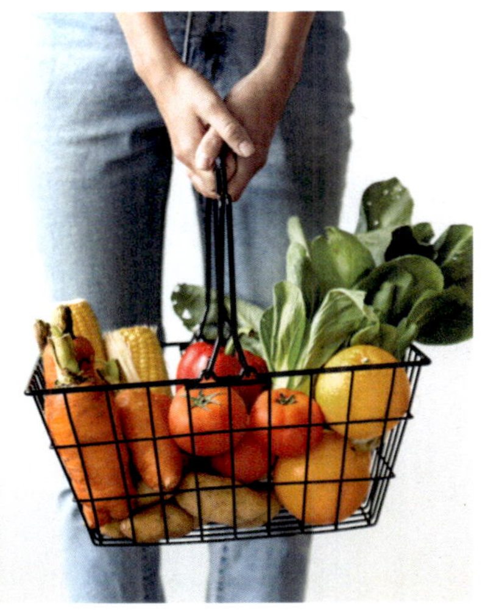

2.

Shop regularly so you won't run out of healthy food and snacks.

3.

Don't worry about calories. Just choose healthy foods to begin with.

4.

Check the label for healthy fats: omega-3, monounsaturated and polyunsaturated.

5.

Reduce consumption of saturated and trans fats.

6.

Try to choose foods with less than 10 grams of sugar per serving.

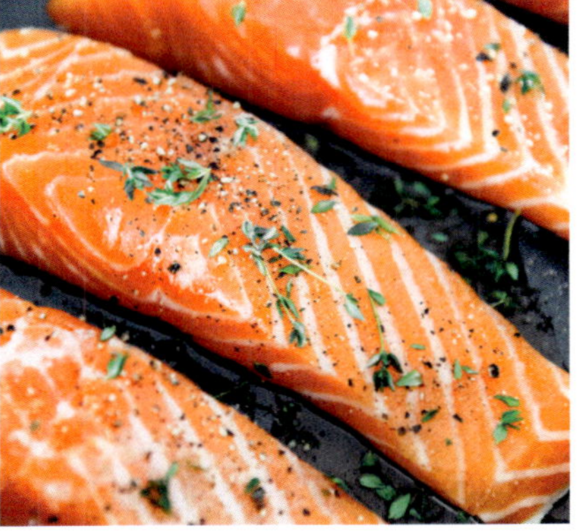

7.

Choose foods with 3 or more grams of fiber per serving.

8.

Watch sodium. Under 200 mg of sodium per serving is a good dancer's guide.

9.

Read the ingredient list. The first three ingredients should come from real food, not chemicals.

10.

Also if sugar is added, it will be in the ingredient list. Make sure it is listed close to the last ingredient if listed at all.

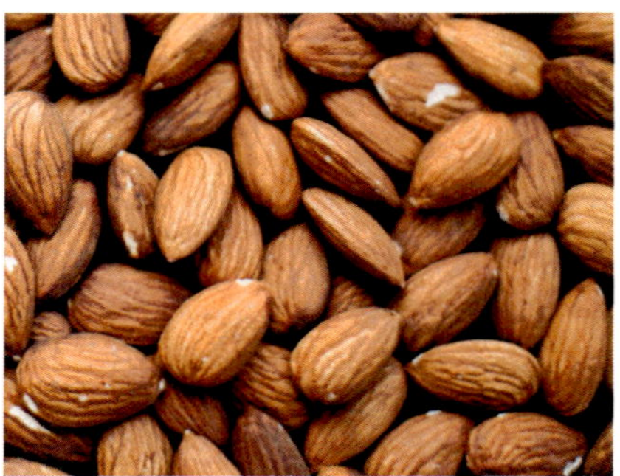

11.

Enjoy your favorite foods often even if they don't fall into our "perfect" categories and ratios. All food can fit.

12.

Use healthy cooking methods.

13.

Invest in a good cooking book or magazine subscription. See appendix for suggestions.

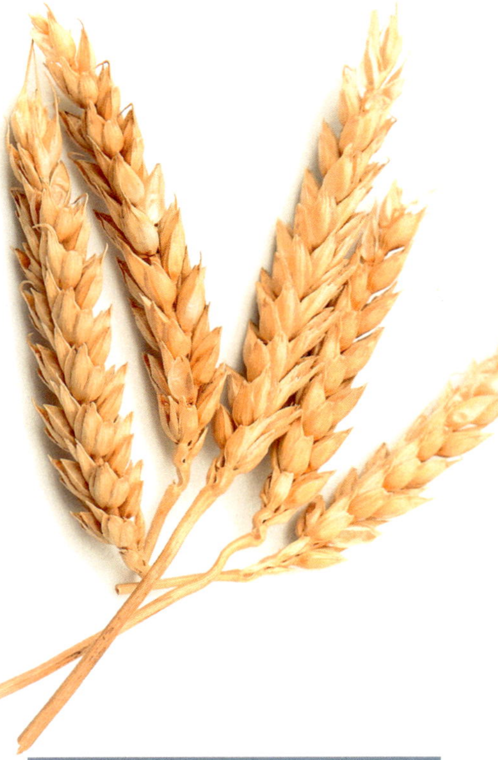

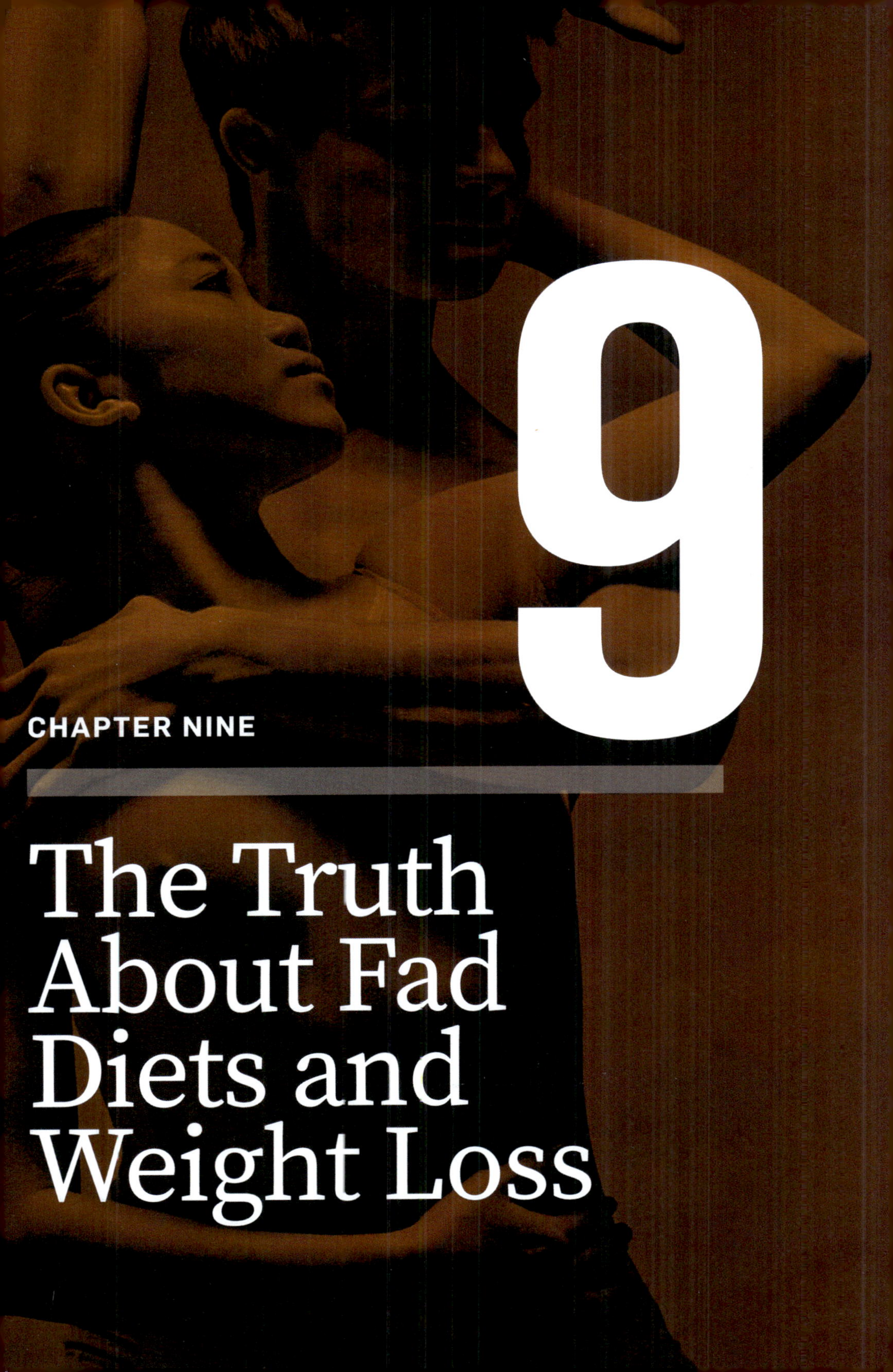

9

The Truth About Fad Diets and Weight Loss

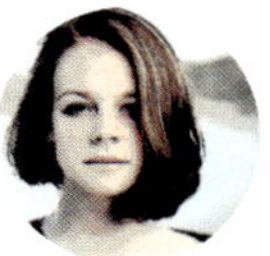 Callie is so confused. Her dance teacher at home in Georgia is always teaching her and other students that it is important to eat a balanced diet to be strong and have stamina. Now that Callie is out of her comfort zone at the summer intensive, she is hearing all kinds of things from the other dancers about dieting, fasting, and cleansing and is wondering if her dance teacher had it right in the first place. She wants to be the best dancer she can be, but if all the other girls are on diets and talking about the latest fads that all the stars are doing, is she missing out on something? The answer is a loud NO! Callie and you need to read on before you make a mistake and go down the wrong path.

Aren't we all hypnotized by the latest fad diet and the incredible claims that promise that fat will melt away? Fad diets come and go. The biochemistry of the body never changes.

Let's review the biochemical truth of the human body: for most of our basal metabolic needs, our bodies require glucose, or blood sugar. We need anywhere from 1,200–1,700 calories per day to provide fuel for basic organ function and cellular respiration. The brain and nervous system need half of these calories. Glucose is the ONLY chemical form of fuel that the brain and central nervous system can use. Glucose is most easily provided from our complex carbohydrates such as whole grains, cereals, pastas, breads, fruits and veggies. It can also be provided by pure sugar; however, diets high in sugar are nutrient-poor. If we do not provide enough calories from carbohydrates on a daily basis, the body can convert some fat (but not much) and protein, if needed, to make the chemical structure of glucose. The process of breaking down protein involves the liver and kidneys, and can create metabolic stress for these organs.

The people who tell you that high-protein diets (such as Atkins, Colorado, South Beach, and Paleo or Caveman diets) are healthy are WRONG. They tell us it is natural to severely restrict carbohydrates and in theory thereby burn fat and protein for fuel. NOTHING COULD BE FURTHER FROM THE TRUTH. And especially for dancers!

In addition to these high-protein diets, there are diets out there that tell you that food combining is the key to health and weight loss. These diets tell you that you cannot combine foods like carbohydrates and protein at the same time because digestive enzymes that work on carbs and those that work on protein "cancel" each other out, thereby making food get "stuck" and creating weight gain and toxicity.

This theory is a WASTE OF TIME. Everything in the body is recognized by SHAPE. Digestive enzymes for carbohydrates recognize the chemical structure of carbohydrates by the shape of the receptor site. They cannot recognize a protein or fat molecule because fat and protein molecule receptors have a different shape. You cannot fit a square peg into a round hole. Our enzymes and hormones act harmoniously side by side because they are biochemically UNABLE to recognize each other unless they are meant to work together. Any diet that has you turning yourself upside down worrying about separating food groups is ridiculous. You have better things to do with your time.

The body needs **1,200-1,700** calories per day to provide fuel for basic organ function and cellular respriation.

Diets don't work. That is why there are so many of them. Because most people who lose weight on diets gain all the weight back and then just try another diet. Let's go over some myths of diets and weight loss:

Myth #1:

If you want to lose weight, you should drastically reduce calories or not eat.

Fact: Cutting back more than 500 calories from what you need to maintain your weight is perceived by the body as too drastic and is usually difficult to maintain. When we eat below our basic metabolic needs (see chapter on metabolism), we might lose weight for a little while, but most likely, it will be from muscle loss. Why? The body's need for calories and carbohydrates is constant 24/7. If we are not eating carbs or eating enough calories, then skeletal muscle and dietary protein can be transformed by the liver and kidneys to make glucose (blood sugar), so the brain and nervous system get the food they need to prevent death. Some fats are broken down also on these high-protein/low-calorie diets, but more skeletal muscle is lost than any other component. This is not healthy in the long or short run. The best way to lose weight is to increase your activity level by 300 calories per day and decrease your calorie intake by 300–500 calories per day. (This can usually be done by getting the sugar out of your diet and watching portions.) That should translate into a one-pound loss of fat per week. Most dancers do not need to lose weight. If the scale has gone up after you have just done a summer of dance that you haven't done before, or if you are new to a new dance school that has you doing technique that you have never done before, you will build muscle to support your new activities, which can make the scale go up. That is lean weight. Don't worry about the numbers on the scale. Focus on your health and how toned and strong you look.

Myth #2:

Carbohydrates make you fat.

Fact: Eating too many calories and not burning them off makes us fat. Carbohydrates come from grains, breads, potatoes, pasta, cereals, fruits and veggies (although veggies are mostly fiber and don't give us much energy). Eliminating these foods from the diet produces low blood sugar, weak muscles, and can seriously impair your ability to dance. Eliminate most of the sugar but keep the good stuff in! Think whole grains and whole food.

Myth #3:

To build muscle, you need lots of protein.

Fact: Consuming too much protein compromises our ability to eat all the carbohydrates that dancers need. This negatively affects your ability to train and compete at high levels. Excess protein is simply excess calories, and eating too much protein can make you gain weight if your total calorie needs are higher than the number of calories you burn each day. Everyone's protein needs are different. If you are following one of the meal plans in the appendix or have used the appendix to specifically calculate your protein needs, then you know how much you need. Really building muscle is dependent on a safe and consistent weight training program that adequately stresses muscles over time. In reality, it takes about fifteen grams of protein to build a pound of muscle. That is equivalent to two ounces of turkey or chicken or two scrambled eggs for example. Don't down huge protein shakes in the hopes of building muscle. Weight train safely and add a bit more pro-tein and overall calories and carbohy-drates to your diet. Remember not to over train, especially during your peak dance season.

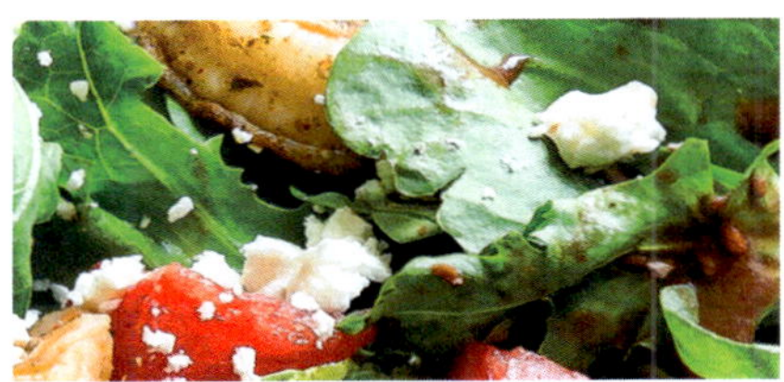

Myth #4:

Fat makes us fat.

Fact: Fat keeps us lean. Fat carries the flavor of our food, so as to keep us happy and satisfied, making us less likely to overeat. The type of fat in our diets is key. All animal fats are saturated fats as well as butter, margarine, mayonnaise, and shortening. These fats produce inflammation, depress immune function, elevate cholesterol, and are implicated in certain cancers. Reduce most animal fats. The fats that will boost immune function, decrease inflammation, lower cholesterol, and may prevent stroke and cancer are flaxseed oil, fish oils, and monounsaturated oils from nuts and olives. High-fat intakes are not recommended, but extremely low-fat diets hurt athletic performance and our health.

Myth #5:

You should never combine foods at the same meal.

Fact: The "theory" behind food combining is that our bodies cannot digest protein and carbohydrates at the same time because the digestive enzymes for protein and carbohydrates cancel each other out. Therefore, the undigested food creates "toxins" in the body. Once and for all, this "theory" is NOT based on the biochemical truth of the body. Carbohydrate enzymes cannot cancel protein enzymes because they have different shapes and chemical charges and so do not recognize each other. They exist harmoniously and do their jobs AT THE SAME TIME. For optimal digestive function, good energy, and to keep our muscles fueled, it is imperative that we combine protein, fat, and carbohydrate at each meal in proper portions.

Myth #6:

We need at least eight cups of water daily.

Fact: Water helps improve the energy and endurance that athletes need and reduces cramping. However, we get fluids from many different sources. Three quarters of a cup of milk, juice, coffee or tea contain fluid, and can be counted toward the eight cups of fluid that we need. Fruits and veggies will also contribute some fluid. Be wary of sodas. Sodas contribute more sugar to our diets than any other food as well as excess caffeine and phosphorus. Too much phosphorus is detrimental to bone health. Strive for at least five cups of water daily. Fill the rest in with other healthful fluids.

Myth #7:

Going gluten-free is clutch for dropping pounds.

Fact: If you don't have celiac disease or a gluten-sensitivity, a gluten-free diet probably won't do much for you at all and especially won't do much in the way of weight loss. Most people lose weight on gluten-free diets because they cut out bread, bagels, and pizza. But once gluten-free bagels, breads and pizzas are introduced, the calories come right back in. Again, for most people who need to lose weight, cutting back about 300–500 calories from what they are eating now and moving a bit more helps them lose weight. Stay away from diet fads and focus on a healthy balance.

Myth #8:

All dancers should do a weekly "cleanse" to eliminate toxins.

Fact: Our livers, kidneys, and lungs detox us every minute of every day. Most commercial cleanses can actually harm these organs and can be very dangerous to health. That is because they often have things like clay or charcoal in them which will force everything out but will also take some good things with it. The colon will be purged but no good bacteria or flora may be left, leaving you with your immune system compromised, and most likely, your digestive balance will be knocked out too. A dance diet should "cleanse" you naturally by providing plenty of whole foods with soluble fiber (think whole grains, whole-grain cereals, breads, pastas, potatoes, fruits and veggies), clean

Water helps improve the energy and endurance.

water and clean proteins (think fish, white meat poultry, beans, nuts, egg whites, unprocessed soy, and nonfat organic dairy) as well as good-quality fats (think omega-3 fats, olive oil, flax oil). Clean your diet out by reducing red meat, sugars, refined carbohydrates, butters, and other saturated fats, sodas, and artificial sweeteners. Do not take pills and potions. Good nutrition works!

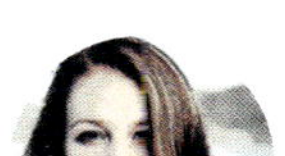

Callie can breathe a sigh of relief. Her dance teacher gave her good advice. She is eating balanced meals, hydrating with water, and getting enough sleep. She even had her favorite cup of tea and two homemade chocolate chip cookies after dinner and knows she is okay. She is looking forward to having her energy up tomorrow for a new day of dance and learning. And she is not listening to all the hype on the popular "diets." Diets don't work.

Myth #9:

You can eat whatever you want as long as you exercise.

Fact: It is all about balance. You cannot out-exercise a poor diet, and you cannot out-diet a lack of exercise. Maintaining a healthy body for most of us is about leading a healthy lifestyle that is fed by real food and prioritizes physical activity. Most dancers do NOT need more exercise. In fact, rest days are critical for your health and well-being. Don't feel virtuous about killing yourself with an extra forty-five minutes of treadmill time just to have your favorite mac 'n' cheese. Dancers burn hundreds of calories per day. You don't have to exercise more just to eat your favorite foods. Eat well 80% of the time, and the other 20% will take care of itself.

Myth #10:

Indulging is off-limits.

Fact: While you don't want to overindulge just because you took an extra class today, it is important for you to eat your favorite foods regularly so that the craving for it doesn't become bigger it should. Dancers can allocate 5–10% of their daily calories to something fun and still be healthy. You cannot live in a food prison. Enjoy your favorite foods often. Slow down, enjoy the flavors and savor every bite. It's good for you.

Review: Chapter 9

1.

Losing body fat is usually accomplished by modestly reducing your overall calorie intake by not more than 300–500 calories lower than what you need to maintain your weight. Increasing your aerobic work to three to four times per week for a duration of thirty to forty-five minutes at a moderate to challenging intensity uses body fat for fuel. For dancers during a busy dance season, the extra aerobic work might be overtraining. Do your cardio work in your off season or just reduce the duration or intensity so that you keep your joints healthy. Do not risk injury by overtraining. Consult a qualified fitness professional and a registered dietitian for what is right for you.

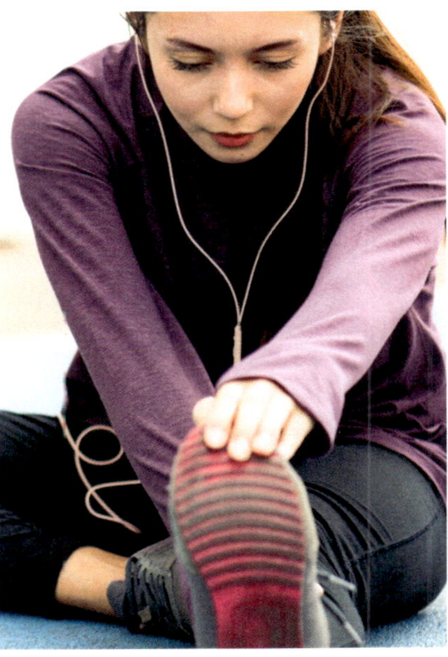

2.

Many dancers ask me what to do to maintain their weight and not gain if they are laid up with an injury and cannot dance. My suggestion is to not ever drastically reduce your food intake in this situation as you need nutrients to heal. Just simply eliminate perhaps your usual afternoon snack, and that should be sufficient to help maintain weight and promote healing while still consuming breakfast, lunch, and dinner.

3.

Diets don't work and most dancers do not need to diet. Fads are fads because they come and go. Consult your doctor and dietitian if you feel the need to lose weight to properly determine how to do it healthfully. Most dancers have a tremendous amount of muscle, and this is often what makes the scale go up. No book can ever tell you how to lose weight. Your body composition should be assessed by a registered dietitian to determine if you are carrying too much muscle or are actually carrying too much body fat. In my experience with dancers, most are not over fat. Thin people are not necessarily the most healthy. See #1.

4.

4. Just because a "diet" is available doesn't mean that it is right for you. If your best friend is "vegan" and does not consume any food from animals, for example, that doesn't mean that a vegan diet is healthy for you. Choosing to eat as a vegan, vegetarian or gluten-free means that dietary intake should be carefully planned so as not to create nutritional deficiencies. I have given vegetarian and gluten-free menu options in the appendix; however, your needs should be individually assessed by your registered dietitian.

5.

Don't be hypnotized by "fake" science. Stay focused not on fads or supplements, but on a healthy diet that contains all foods in portions that keep you satisfied and help you maintain a healthy weight. What is right for another dancer may not be right for you.

6.

Get your nutrition information from a registered dietitian or consult the American Dietetic Association's website at www.eatright.org.

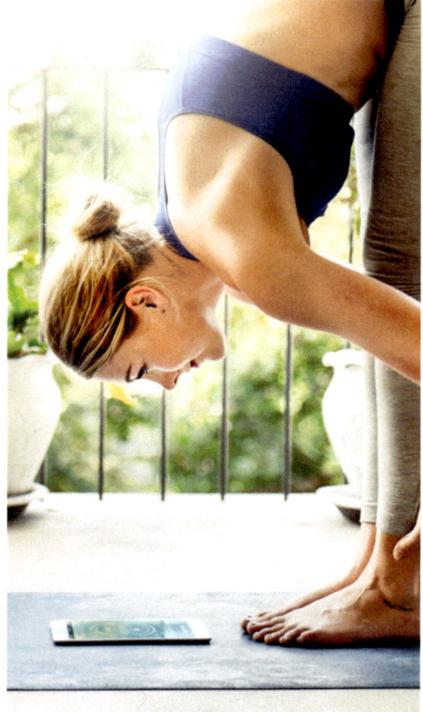

7.

If you are concerned about developing an eating disorder, talk to your parents, teacher, doctor, psychologist, and/or dietitian RIGHT AWAY. These thoughts don't go away by themselves. Get help now.

10

Standing Tall-Healthy Bones and Joints Now

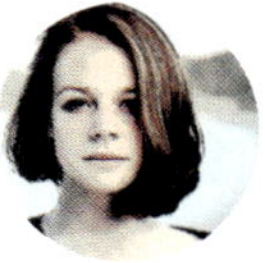

Callie has never had a stress fracture, but her dance mates at the intensive have shared their injury stories with her. She always thought that bone loss happened later in life, but now that she is hearing about the real joint and bone injuries that have happened to girls her age, she wants to make sure she is doing everything she can to prevent injury. Callie doesn't know what to include in her diet to protect her joints. Do you?

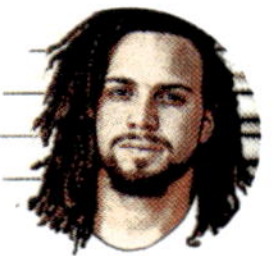

Gregory always thought that bone loss only happened to women. Does he need to be aware of how to protect his bones and joints as well? Should he take a calcium supplement? Do you wonder about this too?

Isn't osteoporosis, the bone-weakening disease, something that happens in old age? Why should you, a young, healthy teenage dancer, be worried about bone health now?

We all have hopes for a long and healthy dance career, but many of us are not aware that we can lose bone now in our teens and twenties. What you do NOW in terms of diet, lifestyle, and exercise sets the stage for bone health and injury prevention for the rest of your life. This is because you are laying down the most bone in your teen years now. Going into your twenties and thirties and beyond with strong bones can almost assure you that you will not suffer stress fractures and other related injuries.

What causes bone loss? We don't know the exact cause of the disease, but we do understand somewhat how it develops. Bone is living tissue, and it never stops growing. Think of your bones as a construction site. Cells called osteoclasts are made from bone marrow cells, and they act like the demolition team. They are responsible for tearing bone down.

We begin developing our skeleton before we are born. This continues through our life cycle. We lay down the most bone (when osteoblasts are very busy) during our teen years and early twenties. Until the age of thirty, a person normally builds more bone than is broken down. If we are not supplying bones with calcium from our diets, with vitamin D, and other minerals, we can easily have weakened bones as early as in our twenties.

Let's look at the overall risk factors and then go into dietary specifics for healthy bones and joints:

Several risk factors increase risk for bone loss:

1. Gender: women are about four times more likely to develop this disease. This is because women generally have less bone mass than men. However, men can also lose bone.

2. Age: everyone loses some bone as we get older.

3. Inactivity: this is NOT a problem for any dancer. In fact, the opposite may be true. Dancers may be too active. Watch excessive cross training and plan regular rest days in each week. Prioritize sleep as that is when growth hormone is stimulated. NEVER take hormones unless your doctor and health team have determined that you need them.

4. Smoking: nicotine in cigarettes prevents osteoblasts from building bone.

5. Alcohol: heavy alcohol use is linked to low bone mass.

Key Note:

Osteoclasts are stimulated by immune disorders like arthritis, lupus, diabetes, multiple sclerosis, depression, inactivity, a nutrient-poor diet, steroid drugs and low estrogen, testosterone, and growth hormone levels. If you are very underweight and have too little body fat, your natural hormone levels may be low. Strive for a healthy weight for your height and a healthy amount of body fat. Being too lean is NOT good for bone health. An osteoblast is a bone-building cell. These cells act like the construction team. They are stimulated by adequate hormone levels (estrogen, testosterone, and growth hormone), isoflavones from soy foods, vitamin D, and proper exercise. Bones are also a major storehouse for minerals like calcium, magnesium, and phosphorus. We must make sure that our diets provide these nutrients in the proper amounts.

6. Hormones: loss of your monthly period and being too thin may accelerate bone loss. Always get a yearly checkup with your doctor and discuss ways to regulate your monthly cycle. This is a medical issue and should be taken seriously.

7. Sodium: diets high in salt make us excrete calcium.

8. High-protein, low-carbohydrate diets: high-protein intake makes our blood very acidic, which makes us excrete calcium and contributes to bone loss.

9. Family history: the tendency to develop osteoporosis can be passed from generation to generation, but this is not absolute.

10. Chronic low intake of calcium and other nutrients.

11. If you do not get a monthly period, your body fat may be too low, which can weaken bone.

So how do we get enough calcium from our diets? First, know how much you need. Teens should aim to consume at least 1,300 mg per day from food and/or supplement. How can you do this? If you can, consume at least 3 servings of low or nonfat dairy products each day. Each serving of dairy will provide 300 mg of calcium. You can make the rest up with nondairy sources, such as broccoli, kale, tofu, and almonds. Some cereals such as Total will give you another 250 mg of calcium. Calcium-fortified orange juice will give you another 300 mg. If you take a calcium supplement, remember to take either calcium carbonate or citrate, as these forms are the most absorbable. Also remember that you cannot absorb more than 500 mg of calcium at any one time, so space your food and supplements throughout the day.

Vitamin D acts like a GPS system for calcium. Vitamin D directs the calcium from your food or supplement into your bones and teeth. You should get at least 200–400 IU's of D per day if you are fifty or younger. Sources include fortified dairy foods, fortified almond or soy milks, supplements and sunshine. Our bodies make vitamin D from our skin being exposed to sunlight ten to fifteen minutes two to three times per week.

Although bones need phosphorus, too much of it will prevent the body from using calcium correctly. If you drink three to four 12-ounce cola drinks daily or are consuming too much protein, as in high-protein, low-carbohydrate diets, you may be getting too much phosphorus. Phosphorus is found in meats, poultry, fish, nuts, beans, and dairy products. Adequate but not excessive protein intake is key.

Magnesium is also needed for bone health. It is also crucial for nerve transmission, muscle contractions, energy production and bone and cell formation. Food sources include dark leafy greens, nuts, seeds, beans, whole grains, yogurt, and bananas. The daily value is 400 mg.

Boron is another important mineral for bones. We get it through supplements (1–3 mg) or from consuming plant foods such as grains, nuts, fruits, and veggies.

Vitamin C is essential to reduce joint inflammation (as in arthritis) and to help build collagen which makes our ligaments and tendons.

Teens should aim for 500 mg of vitamin C daily. Foods that contain vitamin C are citrus fruits and juices, strawberries kiwis, red peppers, potatoes, broccoli, and brussels sprouts.

Remember that osteoporosis is termed the "silent disease" because bone loss occurs without symptoms. However, if you are getting injured or have already sustained a stress fracture, take a look at your diet and lifestyle: are you eating in a balanced and nonrestrictive way? Is your weight healthy for your height? Do you need to supplement healthfully? You have the power to change your health and your career. Eat right to dance right.

Fast Facts:

All dancers get enough "weight bearing" exercise by dancing. Please be careful with your cross training. While it is important to have a strong heart and lungs for endurance, overtraining by adding aerobic work at the gym or running outside may create too much impact for your bones and actually be detrimental. If you need to train aerobically, do so either in your "off" times like vacation or do some "non-impact" aerobics like swimming or biking for twenty minutes once or twice a week. Remember that if all your activity is making you lose weight or keeping you under a healthy weight for your height, your body may not have enough body fat to make your natural hormones. Get assessed by your physical therapist, registered dietitian, or doctor and then decide what is healthy for you. Being too thin has health consequences.

Key Note:

If you are following a high-protein diet and have eliminated carbohydrates, this couldn't be worse for your bones. High-protein diets change the pH of the blood and make us excrete calcium. If you are following a dairy free, vegan, or raw diet, please reassess your choices as your dietary restrictions may not be giving you all the vitamins and minerals you need for injury prevention. Each person is different, and these dietary choices are not for everyone.

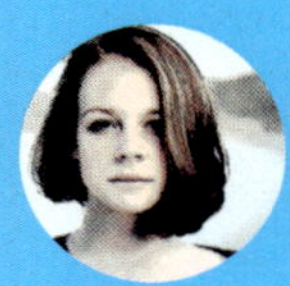 Callie realizes that she is not consistent with her dairy intake. She is going to include a Greek yogurt and fortified almond milk every day. She just got her yearly checkup, and her doctor and dietitian reaffirmed that her weight and body fat were at a healthy range for her.

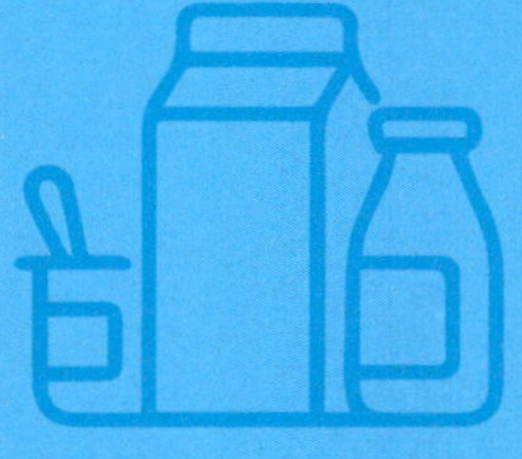

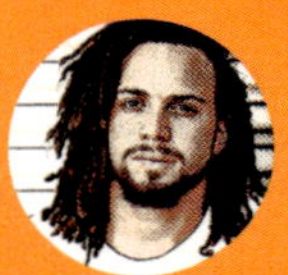 Gregory is a bit lactose intolerant, so he doesn't consume any dairy foods. But he can include a fortified soy milk each day and will steam up some kale and broccoli drizzled with olive oil several time per week. He may even purchase a supplement to shore up his diet but will make sure to get calcium carbonate in under 500 mg capsules, so he can absorb every bit. He now knows that both men and women need to protect their bones.

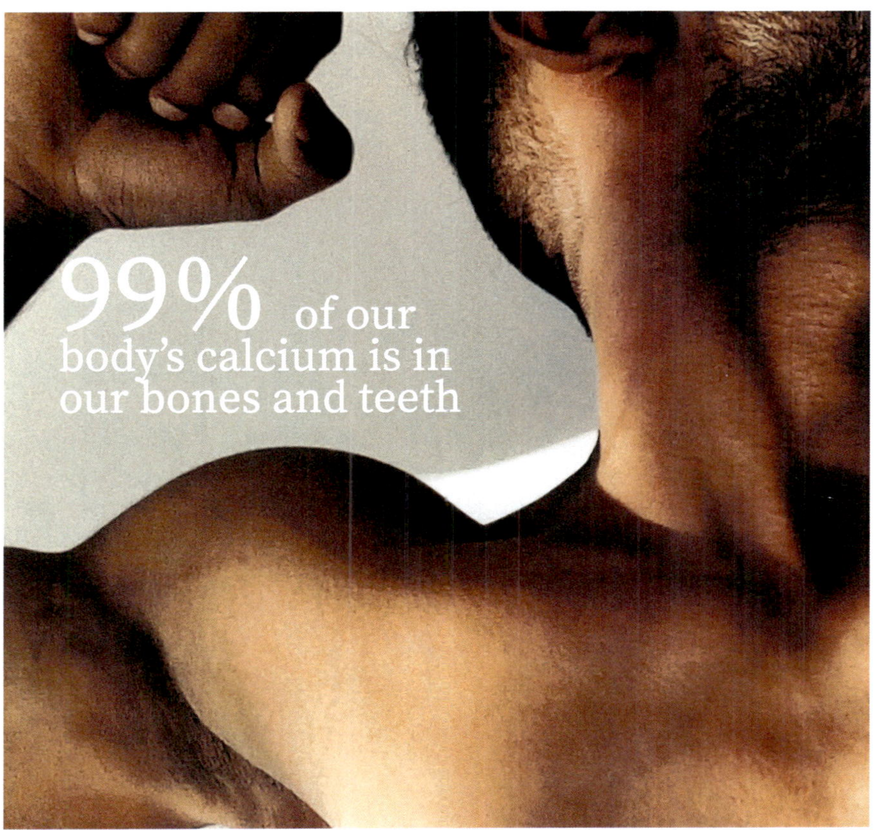

Fast Facts:

99% of our body's calcium is in our bones and teeth. The remaining 1% is in our blood and soft tissues. This 1% of calcium helps our muscles contract, our blood to clot, and our nerves to send their messages. How do we get and keep this 1% of ESSENTIAL circulating calcium from our diets and our own bones if needed? If we don't get enough calcium from our food, our bodies have a way (through the action of the parathyroid gland) to take calcium from our bones and teeth and deposit it in the blood. This is one way our bones can be depleted over time.

Review: Chapter 10

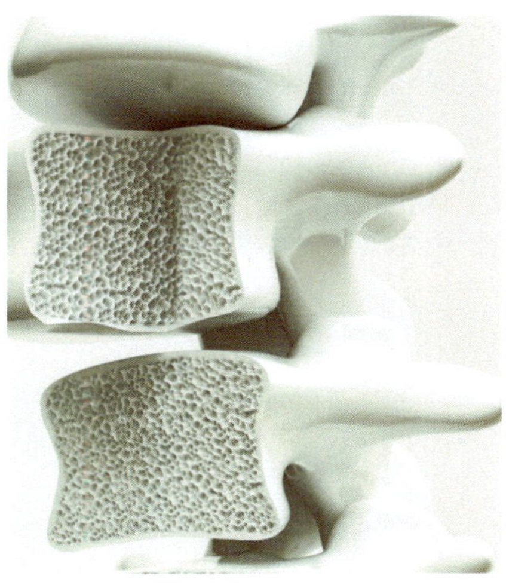

3.

Get enough calcium, vitamin D, vitamin C, boron, and magnesium each day.

4.

Make sure your weight is healthy for your height. (See appendix for height and weight charts.)

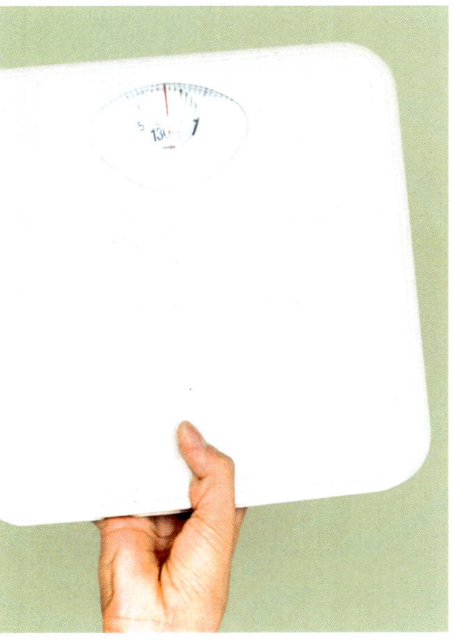

1.

Bone loss can occur early in life.

2.

If you are sustaining bone and joint injuries, the first place to start is to assess how healthy your dietary choices are.

5.

Make sure you have a healthy amount of body fat. (See chapter on dietary fat.)

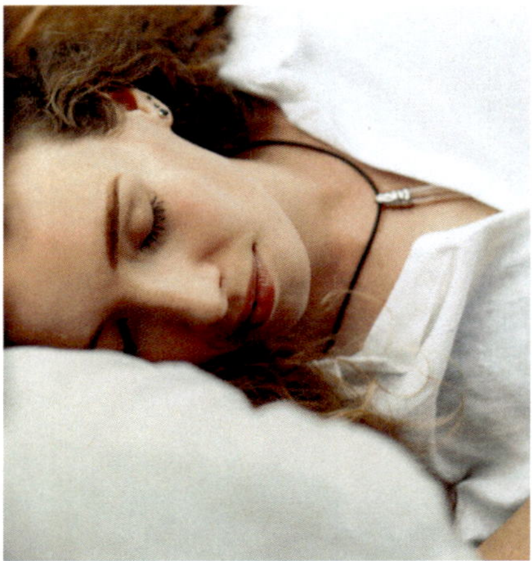

6.

Make sure you include rest and sleep regularly.

7.

Avoid smoking, high sodium, alcohol, and high-protein diets as these weaken bones.

8.

The most absorbable form of calcium comes from our dairy foods; if you are allergic to dairy or have eliminated it from your diet, choose other sources such as fortified almond or soy milks, broccoli, kale, collard greens, bok choy, and almonds.

9.

Supplement appropriately but not excessively.

10.

Reduce inflammation in joints by reducing red meat and saturated fats but include the oils from fish, avocado, olive oil, nuts and seeds, and flax meal.

11.

Don't overtrain. Your joints and body need rest and recovery. Excessive exercise can hurt your bones.

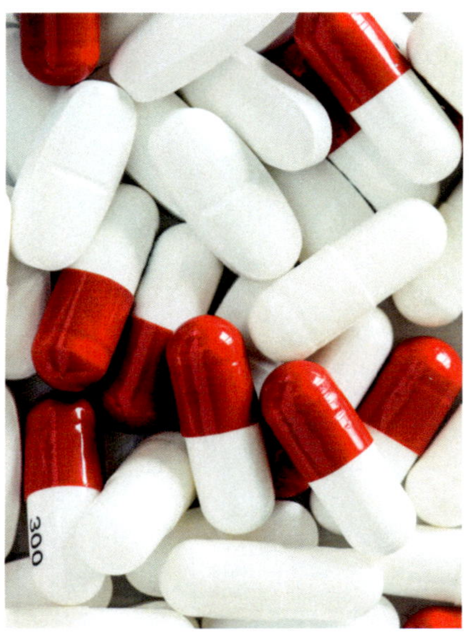

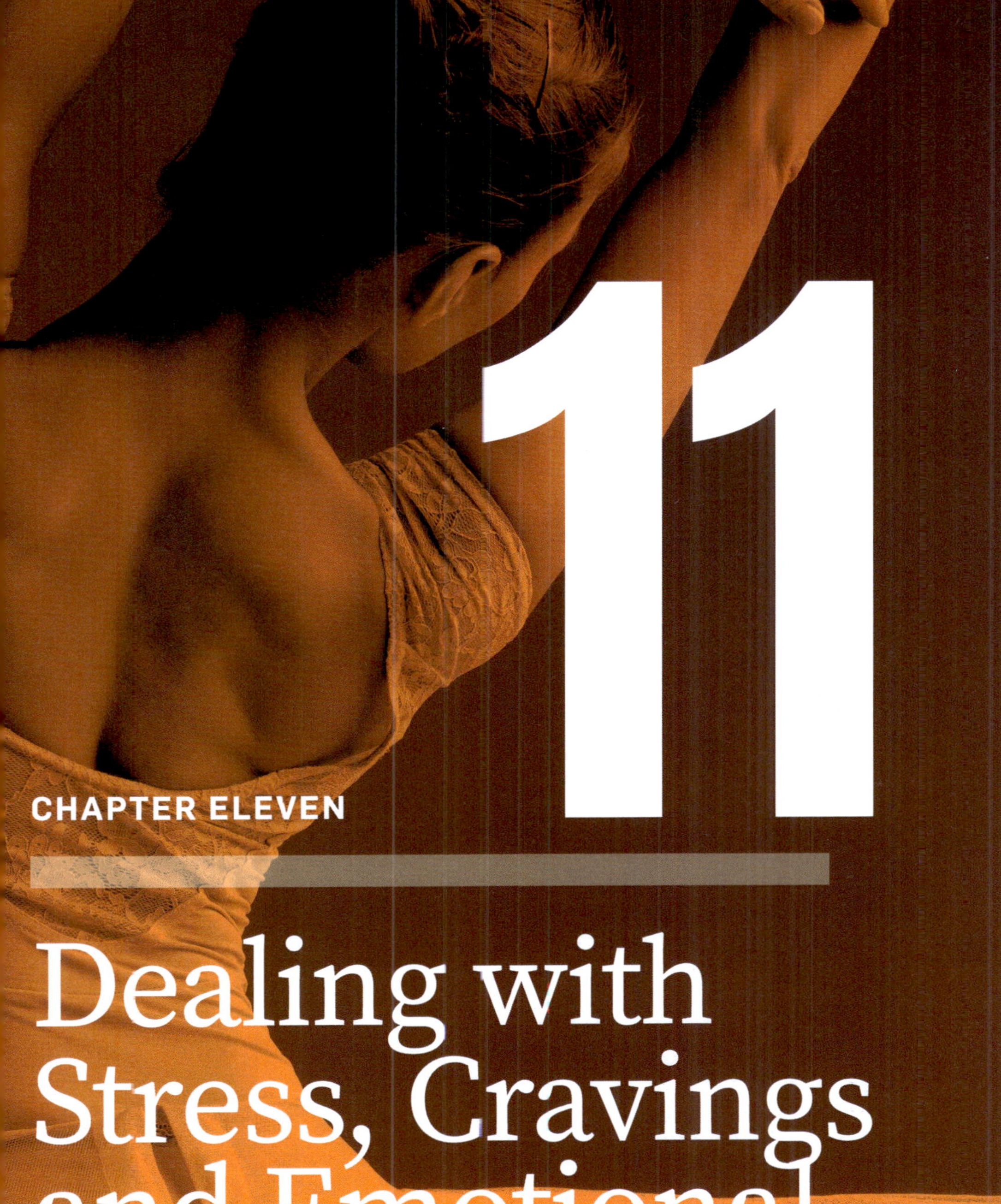

CHAPTER ELEVEN

Dealing with Stress, Cravings and Emotional Eating

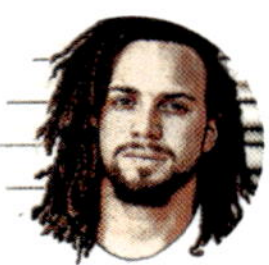

Gregory is enjoying being in New York on his own, but he never imagined that it would be so challenging. He gets up early to take class, goes to any auditions that his agent has set up, and then goes to his survival job later in the afternoon and works 'til 9:00 p.m. All the activities and stress of "making it" take its toll: he often gets tired and doesn't always make the best food choices, especially if he is time pressured. Sometimes, he craves sugar and wonders if he gives in if it will affect his health. Just wondering if he is being healthy is stressful. We will try to ease Gregory's mind and YOUR mind about how to deal with stress, cravings, and emotional eating in this chapter.

Dancers of all ages experience stress, whether it is physical or emotional. You are under pressure to do well, to compete, to be "perfect." But "stress" is a funny concept. What is stressful to one person is not stressful to another. Could stress be our perception or idea of what is happening to us? And if it is an idea, could we change our thoughts and our ways of coping so that we do not get worn down or perhaps use food to deal with stress? The answer is YES. The relationship between stress and individual eating habits is very complicated. Does stress just simply reduce our ability to make good food choices, or does it actually increase our appetites? In fact, it does both. So what stress management techniques can dancers use to help them during stressful times?

Here are some suggestions:

1. Plan ahead as best you can. If you know that you are going to have a full day of classes, rehearsals, family obligations, part-time job obligations, then pack your lunch and snacks the night before so that you don't get caught short. Have extra money to pick up a salad or a small meal if time is short.

2. Get your sleep! Most dancers need between seven to nine hours of sleep EVERY night. Go to sleep and wake up at the same time every day. Fatigue masks itself as hunger. So if you "feel" hungry, stop and think. Perhaps you need a nap or to go to bed early instead of eating a sugary snack. If you need a snack, choose something wholesome: peanut butter on toast, a handful of raisins and nuts, a Greek yogurt topped w/cereal, a cup of low-fat cottage cheese and fruit, for example.

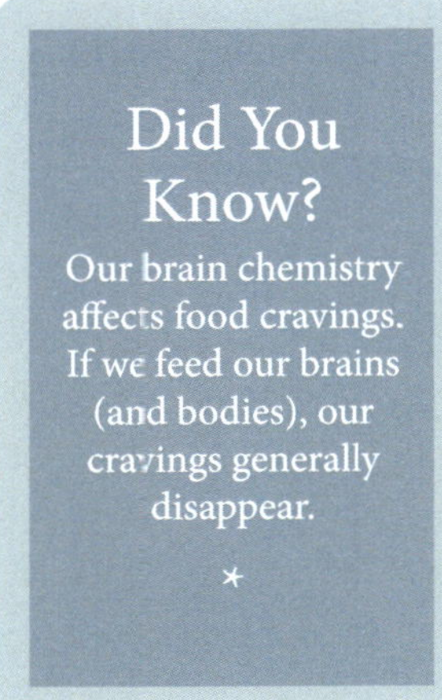

3. Practice deep breathing or meditation. Slow things down and begin to notice if you are eating in response to your tummy being empty or in response to stress or uncomfortable emotions. If you are eating emotionally, then write down what is bothering you or talk it out with someone you trust who will be supportive. Cravings usually go away in fifteen minutes of so. Being physically hungry doesn't go away. Eat in response to physical hunger. Deal with emotions by learning and understanding your feelings. This may take some professional help.

4. Eat in a balanced way and don't skip meals. Low blood sugar can make you nervous and reduce your ability to make healthy food choices and handle stress.

5. Learn to say no. If helping your friend move, for example, means that you will be up until 2:00 a.m. after putting in a full day of classes and dance, this may put you over the top in terms of sleep loss and stress. Having healthy boundaries and knowing what you can and cannot handle will greatly reduce your stress.

6. Take good care of yourself. Do nice things for yourself like reading a good book, talking with a good friend, enjoying your family, taking a leisurely walk and being in nature, listening to your favorite music, giving yourself "down" time to relax on a regular basis, etc. Caring for yourself in a nonfood-related way will take the "charge" off food as a stress release or a "reward."

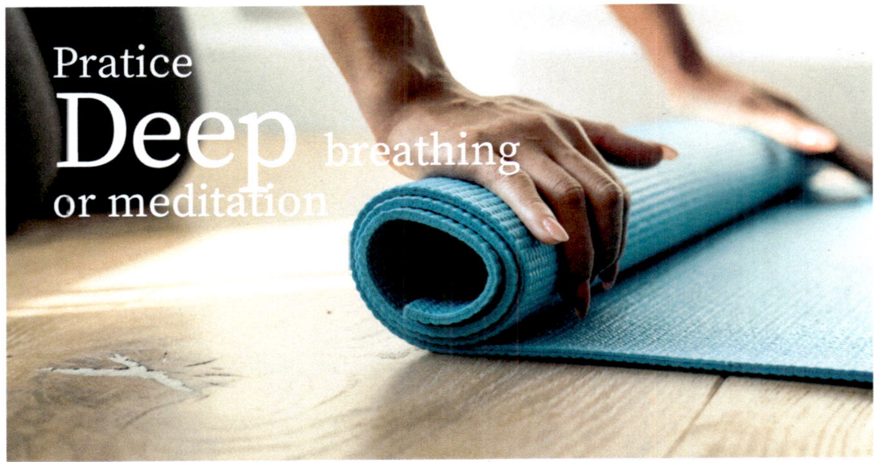

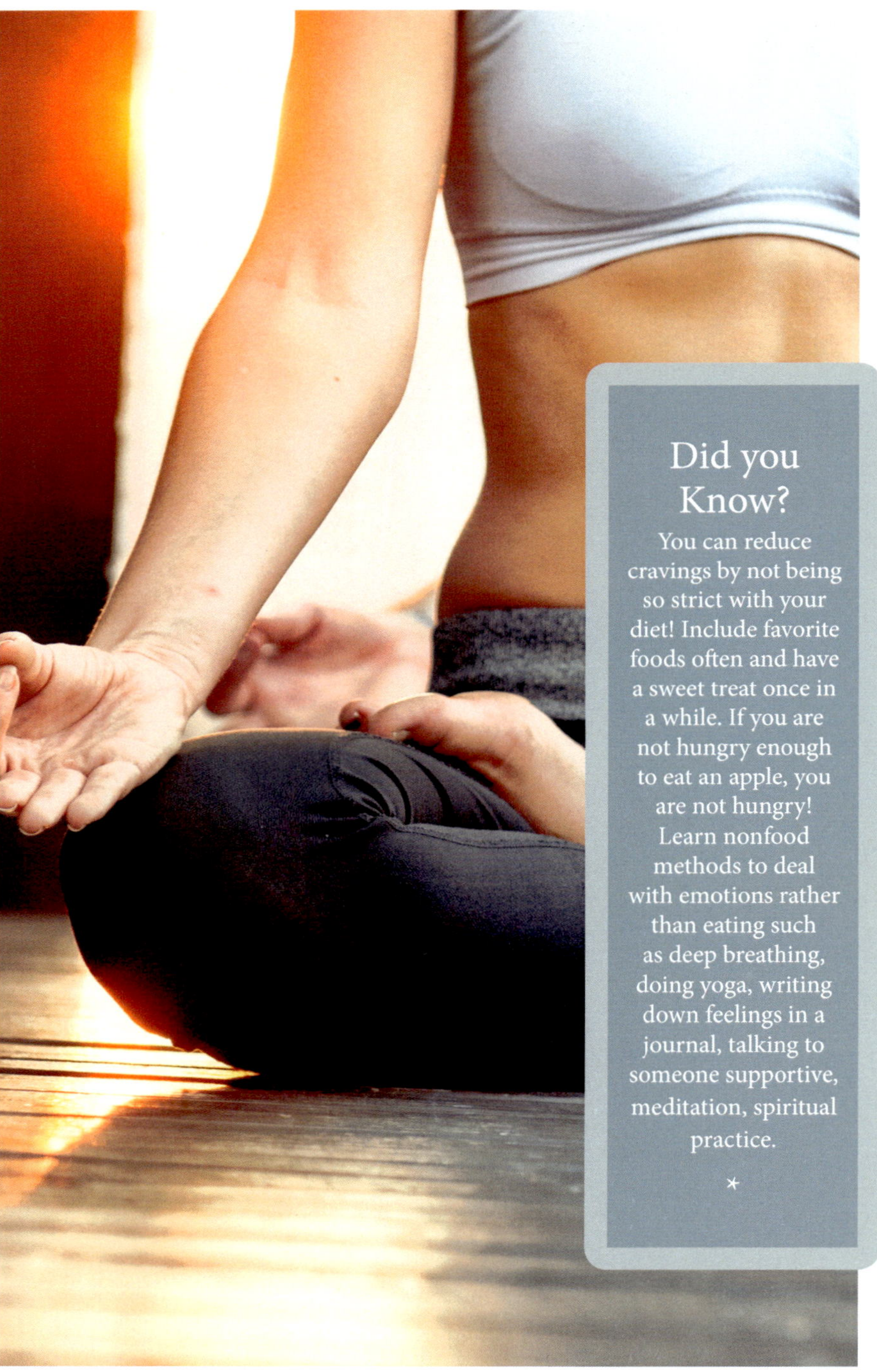

Did you Know?

You can reduce cravings by not being so strict with your diet! Include favorite foods often and have a sweet treat once in a while. If you are not hungry enough to eat an apple, you are not hungry! Learn nonfood methods to deal with emotions rather than eating such as deep breathing, doing yoga, writing down feelings in a journal, talking to someone supportive, meditation, spiritual practice.

*

7. Everyone experiences stress. If you can keep perspective by finding the good or the humor in a situation, it can reduce the experience of stress.

Many of my dance students ask me about food cravings which seem to pop up especially during stressful times. We will discuss them and see that everyone experiences cravings. Cravings are normal.

The chemical hormones in our brain determine what we "crave." Erratic eating or eliminating food groups can really throw us off balance. To know how cravings are created, we have to know how they behave and why.

Here is your list:

Brain Chemical Body Signal	Serotonin	Dopamine	Endorphins	Norepinephrine
	Serotonin is a brain chemical that produces the following: Satiety Sleepiness Reduced stress Mood stability Calmness	Dopamine is a brain chemical that helps with the following: Energy Concentration Alertness Productivity	Endorphins help us feel: Reduced pain Mood stability Reduced stress Euphoria	Norepinephrine is a brain chemical that produces: Alertness Increased blood pressure Increased carbohydrate appetite
Food Component That Increases Its Corresponding Brain Chemical	Sugar Starchy carbohydrates — Serotonin is decreased with low blood sugar, especially in the morning, so if we don't eat carbohydrates or skip breakfast, we will not feel calm or have a stable mood.	Protein — If we do not include a good source of protein each time we eat our energy, concentration and productivity will suffer.	Fat/Sugar — Decreased in dieting and starvation. If we want to feel good, we must include some good-quality fat in our meal (avocado, nuts, olive oil, or fish oil). Also we must never restrict calories below maintenance needs, or we will feel stressed.	Elevated with low blood sugar, STRESS, and is higher in the morning. If we skip breakfast, we may crave carbs or sugar. This may be one reason we crave sugar when stressed: increased norepinephrine levels might be the cause. Another reason to practice stress reduction techniques.

How do you make sense of this? We want to have even levels of serotonin, dopamine, and endorphins to help us feel a sense of calm, be productive and alert, and to have energy. In order to do this, the dancer must have consistent intakes of carbohydrates, proteins and fats every time they eat. If you are skipping meals and snacks, and not eating in a balanced way, the stress hormone norepinephrine will be elevated, thereby increasing your sugar cravings. Take home message for dancers:

1. Never skip breakfast.

2. Always include a good-quality carbohydrate with protein and a healthy fat for a stable mood and good energy.

3. Keeping your blood sugar even by eating well and practicing stress reduction can help reduce cravings.

4. If you want to give in to a craving, you can do so. Just have a normal portion of whatever you are craving and wait fifteen minutes before you "eat the whole thing." If you want more, have a small serving of it. Just slow down and pay attention to how you feel before you overeat and make yourself miserable. If you are not hungry enough for an apple, you are not physically hungry. Practice nonfood-related ways to deal with stress.

5. Eat your favorite foods often and have a treat regularly, so you don't feel like you are deprived.

6. Don't diet! Calorie restriction can cause cravings. If you need to lose weight, a small change in diet and a slight increase in exercise may be all that is needed. Don't decide this on your own. See your doctor and dietitian to be safe. See chapter on fad diets.

7. Get enough sleep. Sleep deprivation will prevent you from dancing well and may promote sugar cravings.

8. Drink enough water. Dehydration may make you feel hungry.

9. Be good to yourself. Self-care with healthy food, proper rest, fun nondance-related activities that can reduce stress like seeing a movie or reading a good book, and a healthy support system from family, friends, and teachers can help you stay on track.

10. Recognize the difference between "heart hunger" and "stomach hunger." If you are not hungry enough to eat an apple, you are not "stomach hungry." Construct different ways to feed your emotional hunger other than food: meditate, go for a walk, read a book, journal, talk to a supportive family member or friend, take a warm bath, listen to music.

11. Cravings generally pass in fifteen minutes or so if you don't give in to them.
If you do, choose a small portion of what you crave, eat it slowly, enjoy it,
and wait fifteen minutes before you eat the whole thing! You will probably be
satisfied and not need to overeat to deal with feelings or emotions. Practice
patience with yourself. Habits take time to change.

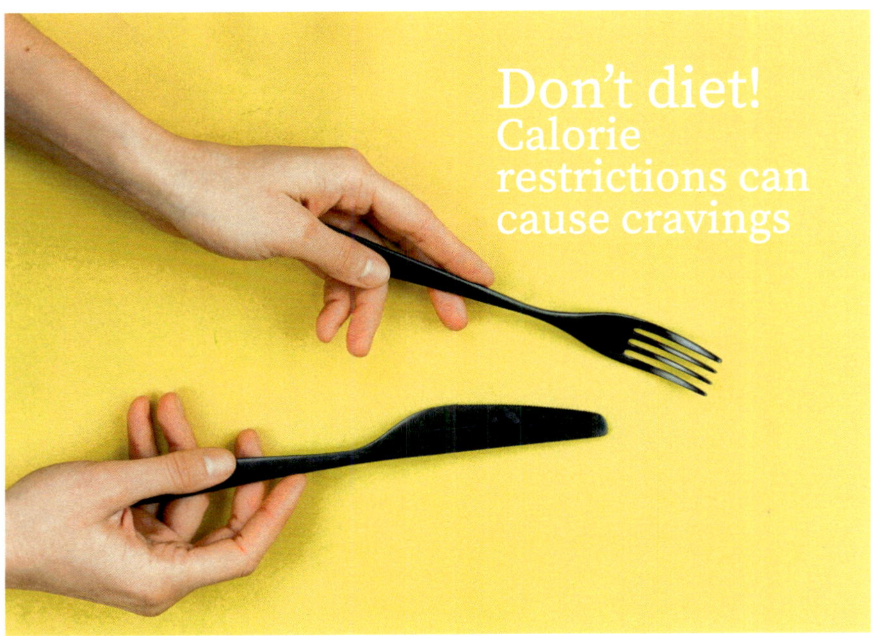

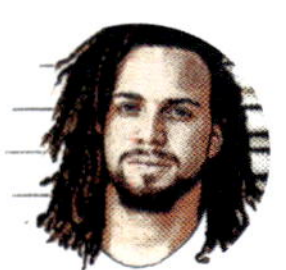

Gregory is so relieved about his health. From now
on, he is going to bring healthy food with him like
a peanut butter and jelly sandwich, fresh fruit,
a low-fat string cheese and cut up peppers and
carrots to munch on during a busy day. He now knows that
a little sweet treat from time to time will not be detrimental.
He can slow down and enjoy his favorite banana nut bread
and not feel guilty. He will try to deal with his stress level
by making sure he has down time every week to just relax!
See the appendix for tips on "creating a sacred
space" to meditate and destress.

Review: Chapter 11

1.

Discipline worry and decrease your stress level by doing the following exercise, originally developed by Thomas Borkovec, PhD of the University of Pennsylvania:

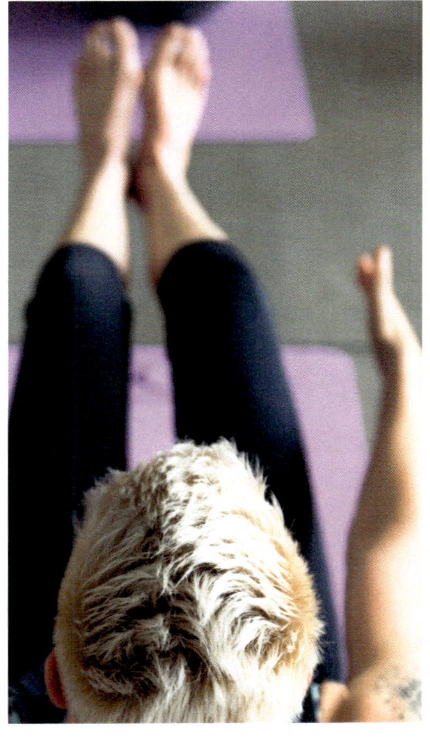

2.

Notice when your worry comes. Don't try to forget it. That doesn't work.

3.

Set aside twenty minutes of uninterrupted "worry time" each day.

4.

At that time, do nothing else. Think only about your worry. After a while, our mind will wander naturally. This natural process helps worry and resentment lose their grip.

5.

Practice this exercise daily until your mental elastic keeps you focused on what is at hand.

6.

This process tricks your stress alarm system into thinking you can handle whatever is happening now—WHICH YOU CAN!

7.

Eat well and don't skip meals. Plan ahead. Always include carbohydrates, proteins and fats for a balanced hormonal chemistry.

8.

Cravings are normal and usually time limited. You can wait it out for fifteen minutes and notice that the craving goes away. If you decide to give in, have a normal portion of what you crave, enjoy it and wait another fifteen minutes to notice how full you are or if the craving went away. If not, have another small portion and continually check in with yourself. Are you full? Are you satisfied? Do you need to distract yourself? Are you eating enough during the day to prevent sugar cravings at night? Cravings are usually a result of decreased calorie and carbohydrate intake. Try to do better the next day

9.

Regularly include your favorite foods and treats so that you don't feel deprived.

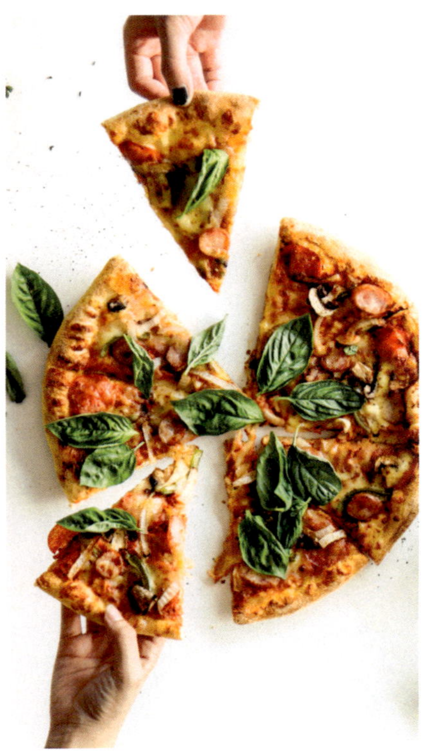

10.

Learn to "feed" yourself in nonfood-related ways: get enough sleep, get enough fluids, eat well and in balance during the day, read books, listen to music, stay in touch with family and friends.

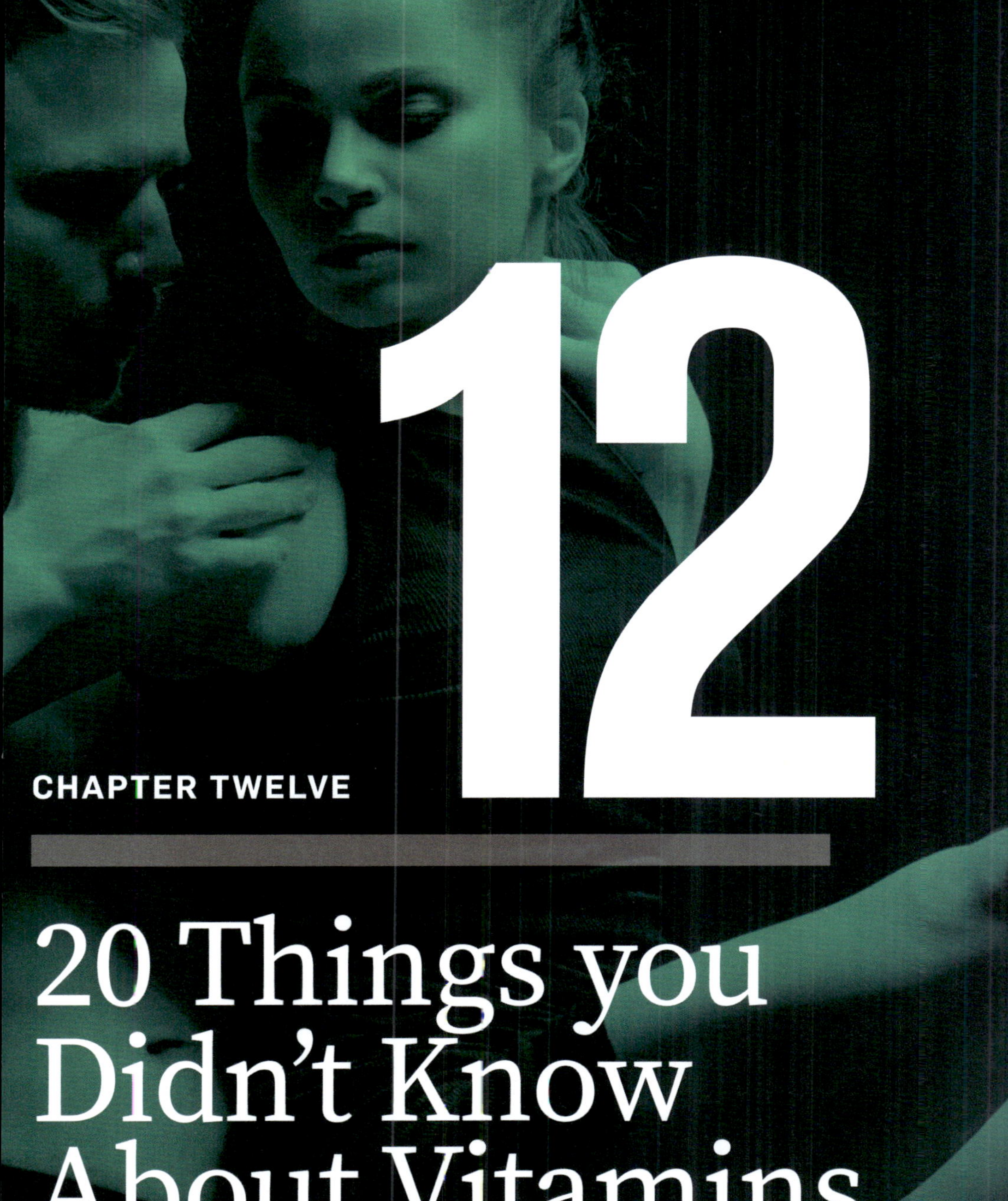
12
CHAPTER TWELVE
20 Things you Didn't Know About Vitamins

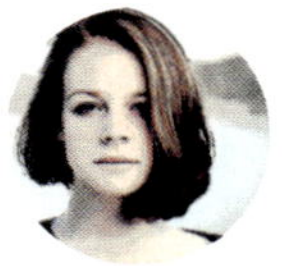
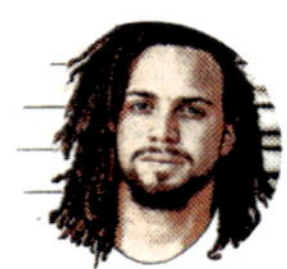

Both Callie and Gregory have heard that dancers need to take lots of supplements to stay healthy. They see their friends buying multivitamins, iron, calcium, and lots of other pills. They wonder what is right for them. Shouldn't you get all the vitamins you need from your food? What is too much? What is essential for dancers?

Question? Do dancers need to take multivitamins to be healthy?
Answer: There is nothing like a sound, healthy diet full of fruits, veggies, and whole grains to supply the vitamins and minerals we need to stay healthy. However, we don't always eat well. Add to that the effects of stress, pollution, and illness and supplements can become important.

TAKE HOME MESSAGE:

Everyone is individual. If your diet is lacking variety or quality, or you are eating in a restricted way such as being vegan, vegetarian, gluten-free or are just not feeling well, I would suggest that you get a regular checkup each year with your doctor to uncover any potential issues, such as iron deficiency or B12 deficiency. Each dancer should get a medical checkup each year to make sure they are healthy. With that said, a good multivitamin may help shore up the weak spots in your diet.

Here are some important tips:

• Read the label carefully to see what you are getting. Many "high-potency" formulas provide only the bare minimums you need to prevent deficiencies.

• Don't pay more for "time-released" or "chelated" products. They are not worth the cost.

• Check the label for how many pills you need to take. You may need to swallow six pills a day to get the amounts of nutrients on the label.

• Never double up on a one-a-day type multivitamin. You will be getting too much of certain nutrients, and that can be detrimental to your health.

• Avoid megadoses that greatly exceed the upper dose limit listed in our appendix. Megadoses of certain vitamins can be toxic.

Fast Facts: Here are the vitamins and minerals that dancers need to be most aware of:

1. Calcium – Dancers need at least 1000–1300 mg daily from food and/or supplements. You cannot absorb more than 500 mg of calcium at any one time. So if you use a supplement to add to what you are getting from food, get a supplement that will give you small amounts of calcium citrate or carbonate (easily absorbed), such as 250 mg per tablet and take small amounts throughout the day. Top calcium-containing foods are low or nonfat dairy, fortified almond and soy milks, dark greens like kale and broccoli, almonds, and fortified orange juice.

2. Vitamin D – Dancers should shoot for 400 IU daily from food and/or supplements. Our bodies make vitamin D from sunshine, so get a little fresh air and sun a few times per week. Your doctor can do a simple blood test to tell if you are low in this vitamin, making it easier to know how to supplement. This vitamin can be toxic in large doses, so use the vitamin chart in the appendix to check for upper limits in supplementing.

3. Iron – Female dancers over age 19 need 18 mg per day; male dancers 19 years and older need 8 mg per day. The most absorbable form of iron comes from red meat. But if you do not consume red meat, other sources of iron include poultry, seafood, beans, peas, spinach, and fortified cereals and breads. In large doses, iron is toxic. Do not self-diagnose and decide you are iron deficient. A simple blood test will tell your doctor if you need to supplement with iron.

4. Vitamin C – Dancers should consume approximately 500 mg daily from food and/or supplement. Vitamin C helps reduce joint inflammation and is important in healing and immunity. Citrus fruits and their juices are good sources as well as kiwis and potatoes! Too much vitamin C may produce stomach upset and diarrhea as well as contribute to kidney stones in some people.

Quick Tip:

Get most of your vitamins from your food. See the end of chapter chart for ideas.

Remember that many vitamins and herbs can be contaminated with drugs and other substances. If you purchase a vitamin, do so at a reputable store and from a reputable company. Among the more reputable vitamin companies are Shaklee, Jarrow, Thorne, and Doctor's Best. Ask your doctor or dietitian for other recommendations.

*

Here is a list of twenty things you didn't know about vitamins, especially for dancers:

1. Don't take your vitamins on an empty stomach. If you usually pop a multivitamin before breakfast, you may want to wait until you have had something to eat. For some people, taking vitamins on an empty stomach can make the stomach produce more acidic digestive juices than needed, just to break the supplement down. If there isn't any other food to slow down digestion and buffer the digestive juices, the result can be reflux and an upset stomach.

2. Pair vitamins A, D, E, and K with fat in order to absorb them. This is another reason to take your vitamins with a meal. A, D, E, and K are "fat-soluble" vitamins. That means two things: they can be stored in our liver and body fat, but also, they need fat to be absorbed. Make sure you take these vitamins with a meal that has some healthy fat in it from foods like nuts, avocado, olives, olive oil, or other healthful liquid oils like sesame or canola oil.

3. Popping vitamin A in excessive amounts is NOT healthy! While vitamin A supplementation can likely improve immunity in children in developing countries, here in a country like the USA, we have access to healthy food! Again, vitamin A is a "fat-soluble" vitamin and can be stored in our bodies if taken in excess. High doses of this vitamin can increase the risk of cancer and may cause bone fractures. In pregnant women, too much vitamin A can hurt the developing baby. Never take more than 100% of the RDA.

4. The "fat-soluble" vitamins have more "staying power." "Water soluble" vitamins like vitamin C and all the B vitamins will be absorbed into the body when taken with a glass of water, and any excess of these vitamins will be flushed out of the body on a daily basis. "Fat-soluble" vitamins are different. These vitamins can be stored in our organs, so it takes a lot longer to become deficient in A, D, E, and K. Again, try to consume foods rich in A, D, E, and K rather than relying on megadoses from a vitamin.

5.The vitamin B complex (which contains all of the water-soluble B vitamins) is key to a healthy GI tract lining. Why do we want a healthy digestive tract? Because the gut is the seat of our immune system. We want to maintain a healthy GI tract to be able to digest and absorb our nutrients as well as to stay healthy. Who wants to have "tummy troubles?" No one! Make sure you are consuming foods that contain B vitamins and vitamin C. Other suggestions for keeping your digestion in tip-top shape include eating regularly, chewing your food well, not eating fast, drinking enough water, and including foods with lots of soluble fiber like fruits, veggies, whole grains, and oatmeal.

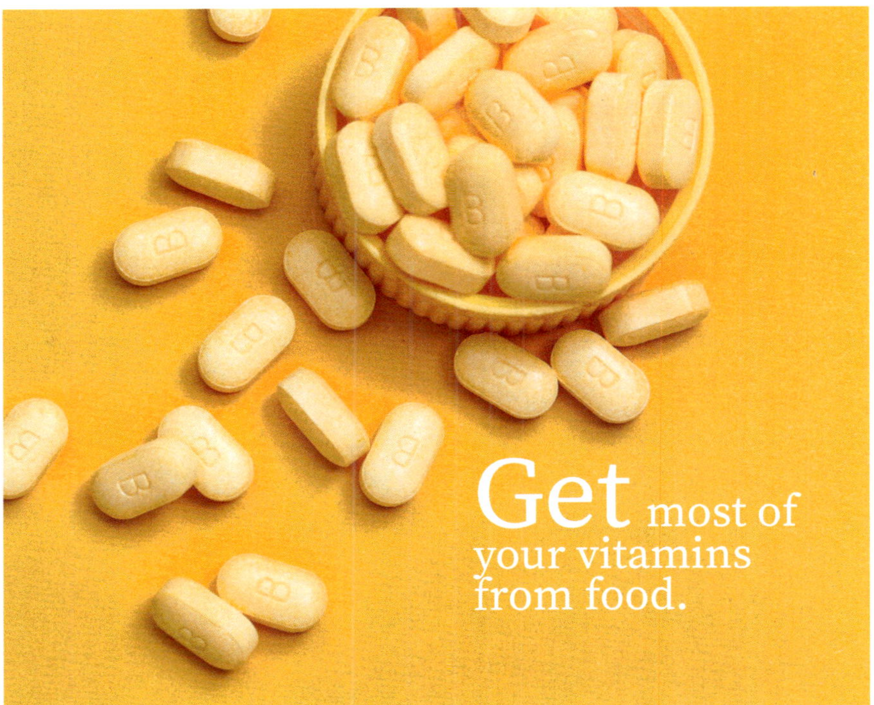

Another tummy suggestion is to eat yogurt if possible for a good dose of healthy bacteria. If you cannot tolerate dairy or have eliminated it from your diet, I would suggest that you consider an acidophilus supplement. This type of supplement provides your gut with the healthy bacteria normally found in yogurt. You can always check with your doctor or dietitian before you supplement.

6. Take folic acid if you plan on pregnancy soon. The U.S. Preventive Services Task Force recommends a folic acid supplement of 400–800 micrograms per day to avoid neural tube defects in the developing fetus.

7. Vitamin C is essential for tissue repair. Anyone who has had a significant injury or surgery should take Vitamin C until the skin heals. Consult with your doctor or dietitian to determine what is right for you. Check the appendix for a list of vitamin C containing foods. And remember, more than 1,000 mg of vitamin C per day may cause diarrhea. In some individuals who are prone to kidney stones, vitamin C from supplements may not be appropriate.

8. Large doses of vitamin C could be a waste of money. Vitamin C is water soluble, which means when you get extra, whatever your body doesn't need will simply come out in the urine. Aim for a bit more if you have a cold, are under stress or live in a smoke-filled or polluted environment. Do eat 5 or more servings of fruits and veggies per day.

9. Vitamin K is essential for blood clotting. Listen up if you are on blood thinners for any reason. For the majority of people, the usual highs and lows of vitamin K in the diet are no problem. However, if you are on an anticoagulant, the amount of vitamin K in the body needs to be kept even. Check the appendix for foods that contain vitamin K; and if you are taking medicine, please have a conversation with your doctor about whether you need to be concerned with the vitamin K you get from food and or multivitamin. We do know that vitamin K is important to help us absorb calcium for healthy bones, so if there are no issues, fill up on those green veggies.

10. Ask yourself if you are sweating out your water-soluble vitamins. Water-soluble vitamins need to be replenished daily from food, so be mindful if you are the type of dancer who sweats a lot in class or working out. It is possible to lose water-soluble vitamins and minerals when you sweat and in extreme weather as well. Don't overdo. Make most of your vitamins come from your diet, and if you take a multivitamin, keep your doses less than 200% of the recommended daily allowance or RDA.

11. Do not combine daily vitamin E with fish oil. We have all heard that the oils from fish are omega-3 fats, and that they are extremely healthy for our hearts and to decrease inflammation in joints. However, these oils can thin the blood. Vitamin E is also an important antioxidant, and we should get some into our diets; however, vitamin E also thins the blood. Too many nutrients that act as blood thinners can make you bruise or bleed more easily. If you take a daily aspirin, this can also thin the blood. Check with your doctor before you combine any of the above just to be safe.

12. Vitamin B6 may help you sleep. This vitamin is used to make tryptophan and also regulates how much serotonin our brain produces. Serotonin is a neurotransmitter that generally promotes feeling calm and satisfied. However, too much serotonin can lower levels of sleep and cause us to wake up more frequently. Foods rich in B6 are chickpeas, salmon and pistachios.

13. Pair vitamin C with iron for best absorption. Some vitamins need a teammate to work the best. When it comes to iron, your body can absorb more of it when you consume something with vitamin C. That is easy to do. Eat a citrus fruit, red pepper, or take some grapefruit juice or orange juice when you are consuming an iron-fortified cereal or a good source of iron such as dried beans.

14. Calcium will compete with iron for absorption. Calcium blocks iron from entering our cells. To avoid this interference, take calcium supplements between meals! Dancers need calcium and vitamin D especially for bone health. Check the appendix out for your daily value. You cannot absorb more than 500 mg of calcium at any one time. So take it in small doses throughout your day.

15. Take B12 if you are a vegan. If you are a strict vegetarian or vegan, then you are not eating vitamin B12-rich foods like eggs and meat. If you fit the above description, then you should supplement with B12 at the RDA of 2.4 micrograms per day. Your brain, nervous system and blood need this vitamin. You can also look for foods fortified with B12, like nutritional yeast.

16. "The more the merrier" is not always true. This one goes for all vitamins, but especially for calcium. We cannot absorb more than 500 milligrams of calcium at any one time. So don't combine your daily yogurt with a calcium supplement that gives you 1,000 milligrams of calcium. It is a waste. Spread your calcium-containing foods and/or supplements throughout your day for the best absorption. Also, too much calcium may contribute to kidney stones in certain people.

17. Increase your vitamin intake after diarrhea. If you get sick and have several days of watery diarrhea, you will excrete more vitamins from the body than usual. It may be a good idea to take a good-quality multivitamin until you are feeling better.

Some Food for Thought:

Dancers want to be healthy and want energy to do what they do best: DANCE! But that may make you more susceptible to believing the hype behind supplements. "Energy" supplements may contain powerful stimulants that can elevate your blood pressure, cause you to become jittery or even worse, make you lose muscle. These can be extremely dangerous if paired with other stimulants like caffeine. You don't need pills and potions to be healthy. Commit to eating well, making time for rest and recovery, and taking care of yourself every day. Food and good training work! Check out the chart for all the healthful foods you can include and enjoy every day to give you all that you need. And check out the appendix to see safe upper limits of all vitamins and minerals.

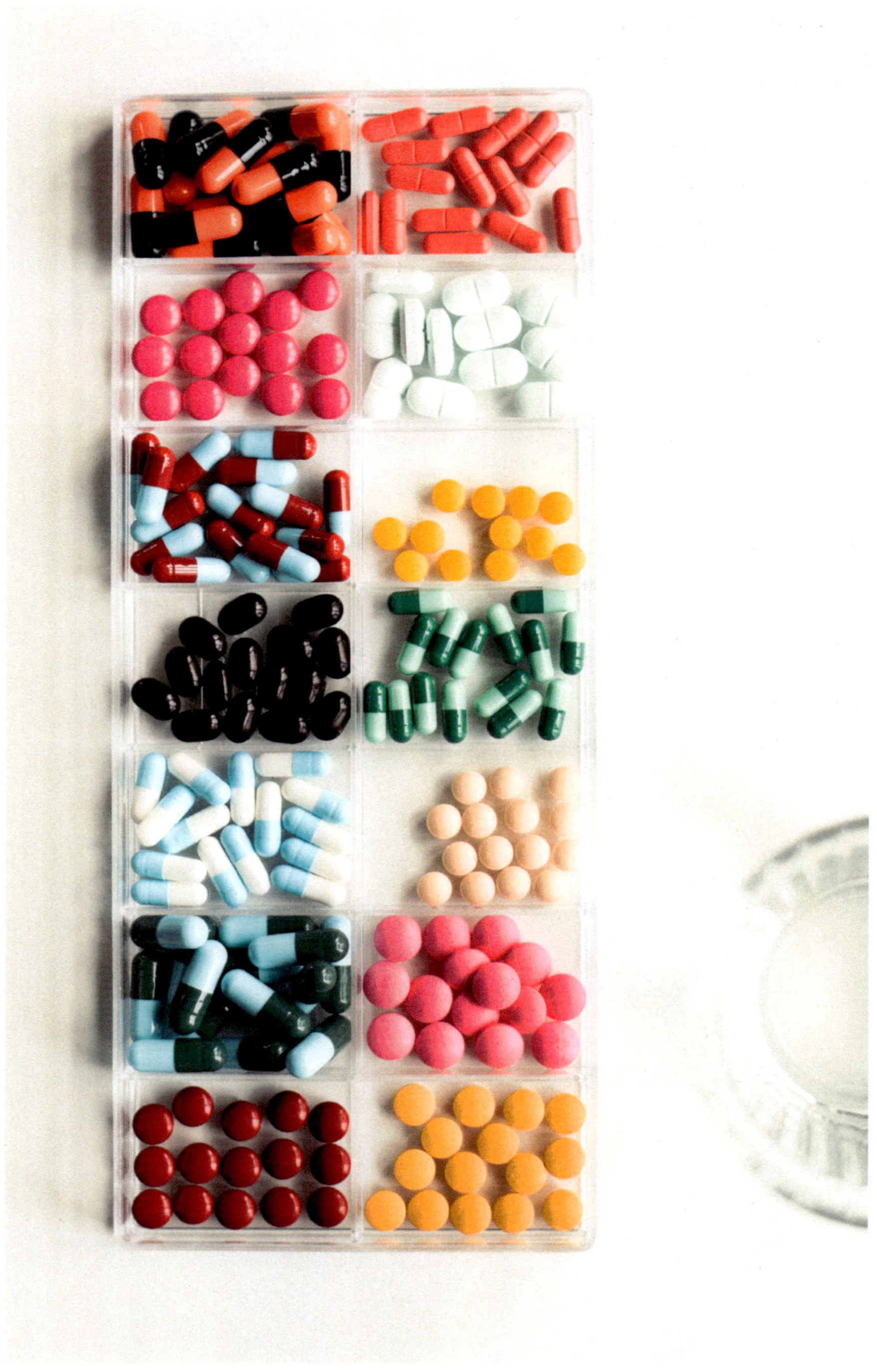

   Eat Right Dance Right

18. Be careful if you are taking an iron supplement. Healthy people taking high doses of iron can experience upset stomach, constipation, nausea, abdominal pain, vomiting and fainting. High doses can also decrease zinc absorption. Check the appendix for dosage and take only what your doctor or dietitian recommend. Excessive iron can accumulate in our organs and cause problems. Don't diagnose yourself as being "anemic." Get a proper diagnosis from your doctor and supplement according to the doctor's orders.

19. Don't mix and match your zinc and antibiotics. Many dancers turn to extra zinc to fight their colds. But if you are taking antibiotics as well as zinc, you may reduce the amount of antibiotic that the body can absorb. Most people including dancers get enough zinc from their diets, so you may not need extra from a supplement.

20. Herbs can also have a big effect on you. You should always consult your doctor when taking herbs. They are powerful and can act like drugs in the body. For example, your doctor will tell you to avoid garlic for up to two weeks before a surgery because garlic thins the blood. And slippery elm can disrupt the effectiveness of oral medications. Consult a qualified herbalist or your doctor before you supplement to ensure good health.

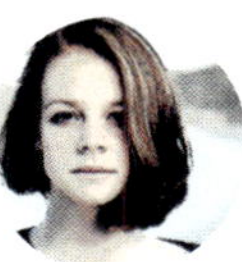

After reading this chapter, Callie looked at her multivitamin and calcium supplements and assured herself that she is taking appropriate amounts of all vitamins. She is going to check out the appendix and use the chart below to make sure she eats the foods that will give her energy and vitamins for dance. Gregory saw that his multivitamin was giving him too much of the "fat-soluble" vitamins, so he will purchase a more appropriate supplement and focus on getting those dark, leafy greens in as often as possible. Perhaps you too will assess all the pills on your shelf and clean things out if you don't really need them. Keep it simple and healthy and don't get hypnotized by "hype."

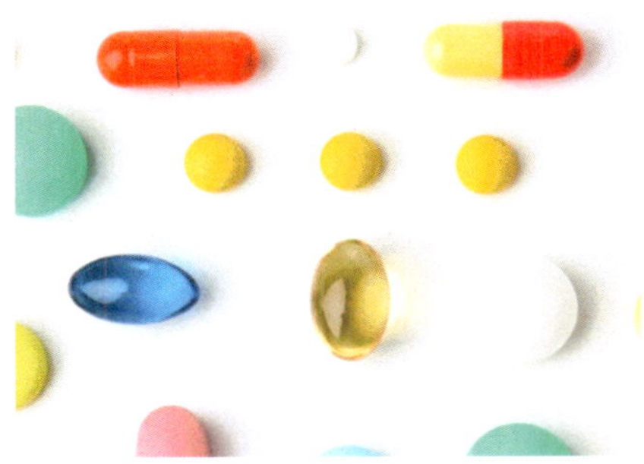

VITAMIN/MINERAL	WHAT IT DOES	WHERE IT IS FOUND	DAILY VALUE**
Biotin	Energy storage Protein, carbohydrate and fat metabolism	Avocadoes, Cauliflower, Eggs, Fruits ,Liver, Pork, Salmon, Whole grains	300 mcg
Folate/Folic Acid	Prevention of birth defects Protein metabolism Red blood cell formation	Asparagus, Avocado, Beans and peas, Enriched breads, cereal, grains, pasta, Green leafy vegetables, Orange juice	400 mcg
Niacin	May reduce cholesterol production Conversion of food to energy Digestion Nervous system function	Beans, Beef ,Enriched breads, cereals, grains, pasta, Nuts,Pork,Poultry, Seafood, Whole grains	20 mg
Pantothenic Acid	Conversion of food into energy Fat metabolism Hormone production Nervous system function Red blood cell formation	Avocados, Beans and peas, Broccoli, Eggs, Milk, Mushrooms, Poultry, Seafood,Sweet potatoes, Whole grains,Yogurt	10 mg
Riboflavin	Conversion of food into energy Growth and development Red blood cell formation	Eggs, Enriched breads, cereals, grains, pasta, Meats, Milk, Mushrooms, Poultry, Seafood, Spinach	1.7 mg
Thiamin	Conversion of food into energy Nervous system function	Beans and peas,Enriched breads, cereals, grains, pasta, Nuts,Pork, Sunflower seeds, Whole grains	1.5 mg
Vitamin A	Growth and development Immune function Reproduction Red blood cell formation Skin and bone formation Vision	Cantaloupe, Carrots, Dairy products, Eggs, Fortified cereals, Green leafy vegetables, Pumpkin, Red peppers, Sweet potatoes	5,000 IU
Vitamin B6	Immune function Nervous system function Protein, carbohydrate and fat metabolism Red blood cell formation	Chickpeas, Noncitrus fruits, Potatoes, Salmon Tuna	2 mg
Vitamin B12	Conversion of food into energy Nervous system function Red blood cell formation Antioxidant	Dairy products, Eggs, Fortified cereals, Meats, Poultry, Seafood	6 mcg
Vitamin C	Collagen and connective tissue formation Immune function Wound healing	Broccoli, Brussels sprouts, Cantaloupe, Citrus fruits and juices, Kiwi, Peppers, Strawberries Tomatoes	60 mg
Vitamin D	Blood pressure regulation Bone growth Calcium balance Hormone production Immune function Nervous system function	Eggs, Fish, Fish liver oil, Fortified cereals, Fortified dairy products, Fortified orange juice, Fortified soy and almond milks	400 IU
Vitamin E	Antioxidant Formation of blood vessels Immune Function	Fortified cereals and juices, Green vegetables, Nuts and seeds, Peanuts and peanut butter, Vegetable oils	30 IU
Vitamin K	Blood clotting Strong bones	Green vegetables	80 mcg
Calcium	Blood clotting Bone and teeth formation Constriction and relaxation of blood vessels Hormone secretion Muscle contraction Nervous system function	Almond, rice, coconut and hemp milks, Dairy products, Canned seafood with bones, Fortified cereals and juices, Soy milk, Green vegetables, Tofu	1,000 mg
Chloride	Acid-base balance Conversion of food to energy Digestion Fluid balance Nervous system function	Celery, Lettuce, Olives, Rye, Salt substitutes, Seaweeds, Table salt and sea salt, Tomatoes	3,400 mg
Chromium	Insulin function Protein, carbohydrate and fat metabolism	Broccoli, Fruits, Grape and orange juice, Meats, Garlic and basil, Turkey, Whole grains	120 mcg

VITAMIN/MINERAL	WHAT IT DOES	WHERE IT IS FOUND	DAILY VALUE**
Copper	Antioxidant Bone formation Collagen and connective tissue formation Energy production Iron metabolism Nervous system function	Chocolate and cocoa, Crustaceans and shellfish, Lentils, Nuts and seeds, Liver, Whole grains	2 mg
Iodine	Growth and development Metabolism Reproduction Thyroid hormone production	Breads and cereals, Dairy products, Iodized salt, Potatoes, Seafood , Seaweed, Turkey	150 mcg
Iron	Energy production Growth and development Immune function Red blood cell formation Reproduction Wound healing	Beans and peas, Dark green vegetables, Meats, Poultry, Prunes and prune juice, Raisins, Seafood, Whole grain, enriched and fortified cereals and breads	18 mg
Magnesium	Blood pressure regulation Blood sugar regulation Bone formation Energy production Hormone secretion Immune function Muscle contraction Nervous system function Normal heart rhythm Protein formation	Avocados, Bananas, Beans and peas, Dairy products, Green leafy vegetables, Nuts and pumpkin seeds, Potatoes, Raisins, Wheat bran, Whole grains	400 mg
Manganese	Carbohydrate, protein, and cholesterol metabolism Cartilage and bone formation Wound healing	Beans, Nuts, Pineapple, Spinach, Sweet potato, Whole grains	2 mg
Molybdenum	Enzyme production	Beans and peas, Nuts, Whole grains	75 mcg
Phosphorus	Acid base balance Bone formation Energy production and storage Hormone activation	Beans and peas, Dairy products, Meats, Nuts and seeds, Poultry, Seafood, Whole grain, enriched and fortified cereals and breads	1,000 mg
Potassium	Blood pressure regulation Carbohydrate metabolism Fluid balance Growth and development Heart function Muscle contraction Nervous system function Protein formation	Bananas, Beet greens, Juices like carrot, pomegranate, prune, orange and tomato, Milk, Oranges, Potatoes and sweet potatoes, Prunes and prune juice, Spinach, Tomatoes and tomato products, White beans, Yogurt	3,500 mg
Selenium	Antioxidant Immune function Reproduction Thyroid function	Eggs, Enriched pasta and rice, Meats, Nuts and seeds, Poultry, Seafood, Whole grains	70 mcg
Sodium	Acid base balance Blood pressure regulation Fluid balance Muscle contraction Nervous system function	Breads and rolls, Cheese, Cured meats and processed meats, Pizza, Savory soups and snacks (chips, crackers, pretzels, popcorn), Soups, Table salt	2,400 mg
Zinc	Growth and development Immune function Nervous system function Protein formation Reproduction Taste and smell Wound healing	Beans and peas, Beef, Dairy products, Fortified cereals, Nuts, Poultry, Seafood, Whole grains	15 mg

**The Daily Values are the amounts of nutrients recommended per day for Americans four years of age or older. These amounts usually reflect the lowest amount of nutrient needed to prevent deficiency. We may need more of some nutrients for optimal health. Check the appendix for the amount of each vitamin/mineral that you should not exceed.

Review:
Chapter 12

1.

Try to eat a healthful diet and get most of your minerals and vitamins from food.

3.

If you do take a supplement, read the label carefully to see what you are getting. Stick to a supplement with no more than 200% of the RDA (recommended daily allowance) on the label.

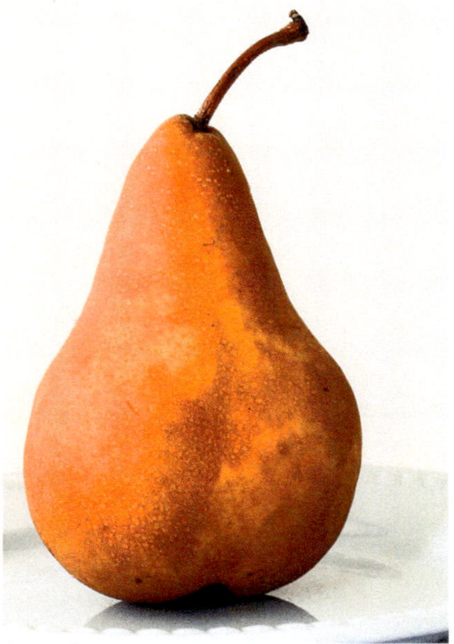

4.

Don't pay more for "time-released" or "chelated" products. They are not worth the extra cost.

2.

Don't take a supplement just because others tell you to. Take only what your doctor or registered dietitian recommend in the dosages they recommend.

5.

Check the serving size. To get all of the recommended dosage, you may need to swallow six pills.

6.

Never double up on your vitamins. More is not better! Some vitamins may be toxic in high dosages.

7.

Watch sports drinks like vitamin water which contains many vitamins. Consuming too many of these products each day in addition to taking vitamins can cause megadosing, which is not healthy.

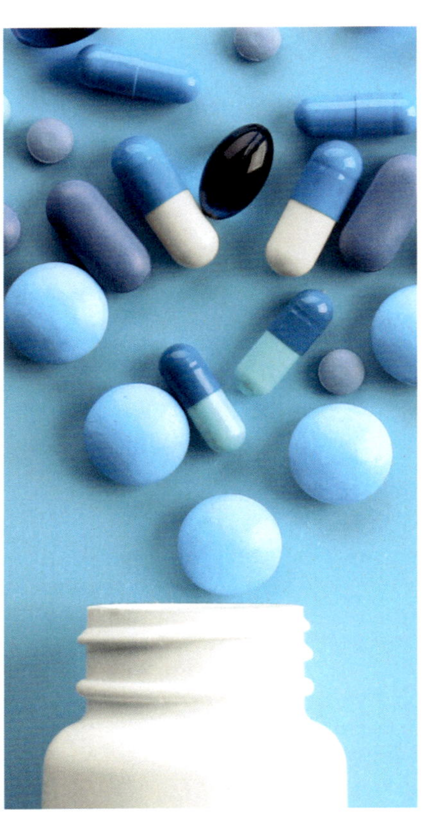

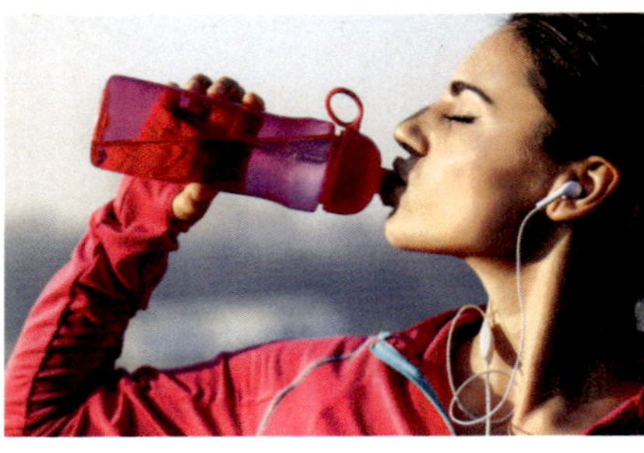

8.

Don't get hypnotized by promises of "stimulated metabolism" or promises of "fat burning." Even if a supplement is herbal, these products can increase blood pressure, affect your nervous system and can be very dangerous.

9.

See the chart on pages 136 and 137 for how your food provides vitamins and minerals.

10.

See the appendix for finding the upper limit of intake for your vitamins and minerals.

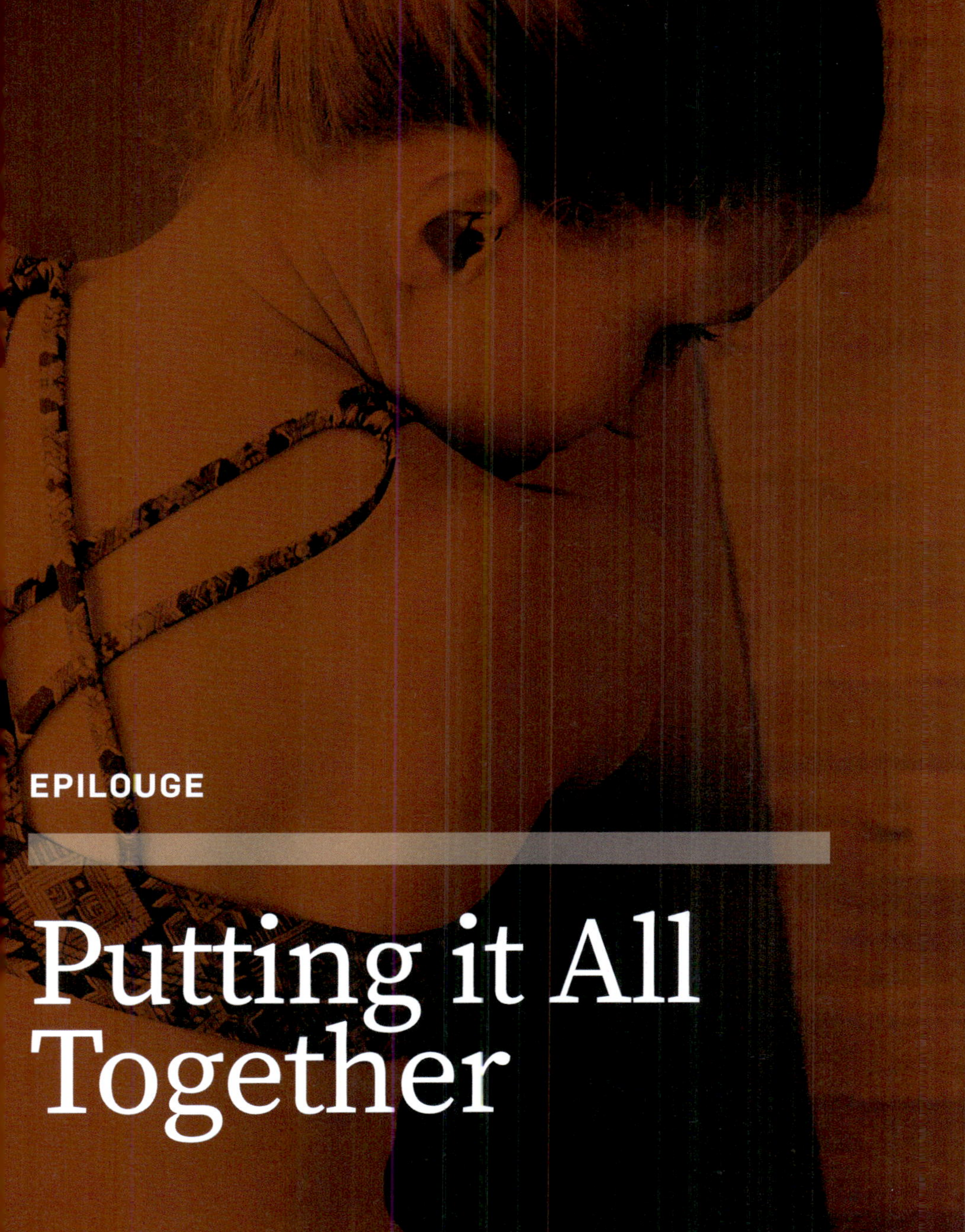

Putting it All Together

• Use this book as a simple guide for nutritional balance.

• Do the best you can each day without striving for perfection.

• Know what is right for you as a dancer by focusing on science and truth, not fads and hearsay.

• Plan your eating day around your dance and school schedule so you won't be caught short. Always pack healthy snacks.

• Make a hydration plan and stick to it.

• Focus on whole foods and don't eliminate whole food groups—be a "flexitarian."

• Look over the menu plans for meal and snack ideas to make sure that you are eating enough.

• Stay away from fad diets and bogus supplements.

• Never focus on the scale as the ultimate guide to health—notice how strong you are, how muscular you are, how strong your immune system is, how much energy you have and how few injuries you have as better signs of health.

• Always get a yearly checkup with your doctor and seek out the services of a registered dietitian. Most health insurance companies cover nutrition.

• Take care of yourself physically, mentally, and spiritually by getting enough rest, eating healthy foods, spending time doing fun nondance activities and generally striving for balance in all things

• Eat Right to Dance Right!

Appendix 1: Calculating Metabolic Rate

The Harris Benedict Formula for Calculating Basal Metabolic Rate
From the American Dietetic Association September 2003, Frankenfield et al
For men: 66.5 + (13.75 x weight) + (5.003 x height) - (6.775 x age) = BMR
For women: 655.1 + (9.563 x weight) + (1.850 x height) - (4.676 x age) = BMR

Weight is in kilograms. Divide your weight in pounds by 2.2 to determine weight in kilograms.

Height is in centimeters. Multiply your height in inches by 2.54 to determine height in centimeters. Age stays the same.

When you calculate your BMR by using the above formula, you now need to multiply that number by the below activity factor. That will tell you the number of calories you need for your basic metabolic needs and what you need also do dance and live. You will get a ball park idea of how many calories you need to maintain your weight give or take a bit. This is NOT written in stone and is at best an educated idea.
When in doubt, eat more.

Activity Factor	Category	Definition
1.2	Sedentary	Little or no exercise
1.375	Lightly active	Light exercise or sport 1–3 days per week
1.55	Moderately active	Moderate exercise or sport 3–5 days per week
1.725	Very active	Hard exercise or sport 6–7 days per week. MOST DANCERS ARE HERE!
1.9	Extremely active	Hard daily exercise or sport and a physical job

Use the chart above to determine the number of calories above and beyond your basal metabolic rate that you need to maintain your weight. (Katch and McArdle 1996)

For example, a 22-year-old male dancer who is 5'10" tall and weighs 165 pounds would need 1,838 calories for his basal metabolic rate. If multiplied by the 1.725 activity factor in theory, this young man would need 3,170 calories per day. That is a lot of calories. Don't ever think dancers shouldn't eat much!

Appendix 2: Calculating Grams of Carbohydrates Needed Per Day

For dancers, experts recommend getting 6–10 grams of carbohydrates per kilogram of body weight. To convert weight in pounds to kilograms, simply divide your weight in pounds by 2.2. For a 108-pound female dancer, that is 294 grams of carbohydrates. (108 divided by 2.2 = 49 kilograms) (49 kg multiplied by 6 = 294) My goal is not to have you walk around with a calculator trying to tally up your carbohydrate servings. I just want you to be aware of generally what we are recommending for a day's intake so that you can make better food choices. If you refer to the serving size chart and calorie ranges in our metabolism and calorie chapter, you will automatically be consuming enough carbohydrates. For those of you who want to be specific, I have created a chart so that you can understand serving sizes and grams of carbohydrate. Refer to the chapter on carbohydrates.

Appendix 3: Calculating Protein Grams

Here are examples of calculations:

To determine how many grams of protein you need based on your weight, you divide your weight in pounds by 2:2 to give you your weight in kilograms and then multiply that by approximately 1.2 to 1.5 to give you the number of grams of protein you should consume daily.

So, for a 110-pound female dancer, that would be 60–75 grams of protein each day. (110 divided by 2.2 = 50; 50 X 1.2 = 60; 50 X 1.5 = 75)

Another way to look at it is if this 110-pound dancer ate 2,100 calories per day and 15% of those calories should be protein, you would multiply 2,100 by .15 and get 315 calories. Then divide those calories by 4 since one gram of protein= 4 calories, and you get 78.7 grams of protein daily. (Multiply your calorie intake by .15 to get protein calories. Then divide by 4 to get grams of protein.)

Appendix 4: Calculating Fat Grams Per Day

How many grams of fat should you consume on a daily basis? If we want 25% of our calories to come from fat, then here is a calculation that you can do:

For example, if you decide that you deserve and need about 2,600 calories per day and 25% of those calories should come from fat, then you would multiply 2,600 X .25 and get 650 calories. You would then divide that by 9 (because 1 gram of fat = 9 calories). So 650 divided by 9 = 72 grams. It is too time consuming to plan out meals in exactly the perfect fat gram ratio. If you just choose lean proteins and low-fat dairy foods and keep your added fat to approximately 2–3 tablespoons (6–9 teaspoons) per day, you will be doing fine. Look at your appendix to see calorie and nutrient breakdowns if you are curious but keep it loose.

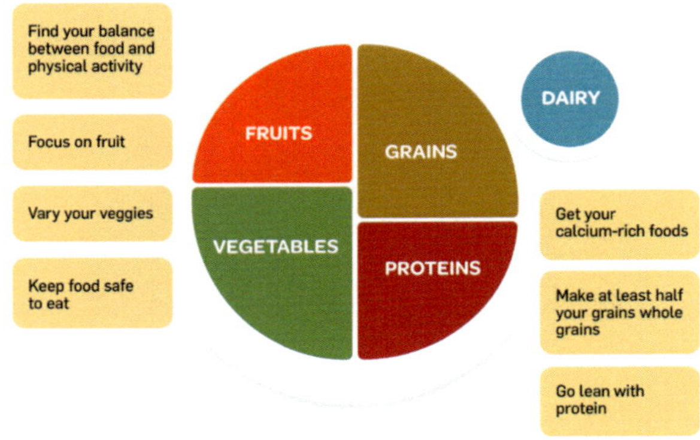

Appendix 6: Resources: Websites and Books

American Dietetics Association, www.eatright.org
Academy for Eating Disorders, www.anred.com
American Psychiatric Association, www.psychiatry.org
Center for Mind/Body Studies, www.cmbm.org

American Council on Exercise, www.acefitness.org
International Dance Exercise Association, www.ideafit.com
Dr. Andrew Weil for Information on Herbs. www.drweil.com
FDA Nutrition Information for Consumers, www.fda.gov/nutritioneducation

Books on Healthy Eating and Cooking That You Might Find Useful:

Roth, G. Breaking Free From Compulsive Eating. New York, NY. Penguin Books, 1989
Amen, D.G. Change Your Brain, Change Your Life. New York, NY. Times Books, 1998
Tribole, E. and Resch, E. Intuitive Eating: A Recovery Book for the Chronic Dieter. New York, NY: St. Martin's Press, 1995

These can be found online and even downloaded:
Brown, Alton. I'm Just Here for the Food.
Bittman, Mark. How to Cook Everything.
Bittman, Mark. How to Cook Everything Vegetarian.
Ray, Rach I. Rachel Ray 365: A Year of Deliciously Different Dinners
Rombauer, Irma and Rombauer Becker, Marion. The Joy of Cooking.
The Better Homes and Gardens New Cookbook

Appendix 7: Creating A Sacred Space

Benefits of Creating a Sacred Space:

• We all have a sacred space within us. However, we can often become disconnected from this inner calm because of the demands and chaos of our outside worlds. Creating an "external" sacred space helps you find that calm space within you to help you recharge and get grounded again.

• Where can you put your quiet space, especially if you live with three roommates? You don't need a whole room. Perhaps it is an alcove or a quiet corner of a room, or just a space with a meditation mat. You could even use a patio or balcony.

Elements to include:
1. Photos of special people in your life
2. Candles or incense
3. Pillows
4. Book of quotations or written prayer
5. Shells, flowers, rocks or plants

Using your quiet space:
1. What do you do there? You can just sit and reflect.
2. Do some meditation or relaxation breathing
3. Yoga, tai chi or qigong
4. Singing or listening to music
5. Reading inspirational writing

If you are skeptical about the benefits of focusing inward and slowing down, give it a month. See if you are calmer and better able to handle the stress in your life. You don't need to spend hours in your sacred space to reap benefits. Even a few minutes a day can help you stay centered and less likely to engage in unhealthy behaviors.

Appendix 8: What to Watch for in a Multivitamin

See the amounts of each vitamin and mineral you might find in a multivitamin or an extra-strength supplement compared to the government's daily value. Going above the upper limits in an extra strength version may not be healthy.

Vitamins	Main Benefits	Daily Value	One a Day	Extra Strength
Vitamin A	Helps fight infections, maintains eye and skin health.	5,000 IU	5,000 IU	5,000–10,000 IU (up to 10,000 IU as beta-carotene
Vitamin C	Fights colds; may help prevent cancer, heart disease, cataracts.	60 mg	60–100 mg	100–1,000 mg
Vitamin D	Promotes healthy bones and teeth; may prevent cancer.	400 IU	200–400 IU	400–600 IU
Vitamin E	May help prevent cancer, heart disease and cataracts.	30 IU	30–100 IU	100–400 IU
Thiamin (Bl)	Aids in energy production; promotes nerve and heart health.	1.5 mg	1.5–25 mg	25–100 mg
Riboflavin (B2)	May prevent cataracts and migraines; helps heal rosacea.	1.7 mg	1.7–25 mg	25-100 mg
Niacin (B3)	Helps lower cholesterol and improve circulation; fosters healthy nerve cells.	20 mg	20–25 mg	25–100 mg
Vitamin B6	May prevent heart disease and stroke; maintains nervous system health. Avoid taking more than 200 mg on a daily basis.	2 mg	2–25 mg	25–100 mg
Folic Acid	Prevents birth defects, heart disease, possibly some cancers.Pregnant women and women planning to become pregnant should get at least 600mcg daily.	400 mcg	400 mcg	400-500 mcg
Pantothenic acid	Builds bones; may aid in diabetes.	*	0–25 mcg	25–50 mcg
Zinc	May help immune system.	15 mg	15 mg	15–30 mg

Vitamins	Main Benefits	Daily Value	One a Day	Extra Strength
Vitamin B12	Promotes nerve health; prevents heart disease. People over 50 and vegetarians should look or formulas that supply at least l00 mcg.	6 mcg	6–50 mcg	50–400 mcg
Biotin	Promotes healthy nails, hair, and nerves.	300 mcg	0–l00 mcg	100–300 mcg
Pantothenic acid (B5)	Strengthens nerves; promotes energy metabolism.	10 mg	10–25 mg	25–100 mg
Boron	Builds strong bones, teeth and nails.	*	0–50 mcg	50 mcg–2 mg
Calcium	Prevents or slows osteoporosis.	1,000 mg	200–400 mg	1,500 mg
Chromium	Maintains healthy blood sugar levels; helps break down fats.	120 mcg	0–100 mcg	100–200 mcg
Copper	Prevents cardiovascular disease; maintains bones, tendons, and nerves.	2 mg	1–2 mg	1–2 mg
Iron	Prevents anemia.	18 mg	0–18 mg	0–18 mg
Magnesium	Protects against heart disease.	400 mg	100–200 mg	200–400 mg
Manganese	Strengthens bones; may be good for the heart and prevention of seizures.	2 mg	2–5 mg	5–10 mg
Molybdenum	Helps the body use iron and burn fats.	75 mcg	25–65 mcg	65–100 mcg
Potassium	May help prevent high blood pressure, heart disease and stroke.	3 500 mg	5–100 mg	5–100 mg
Pantothenic acid	May help prevent cancer, heart disease, cataracts and macular degeneration.	70 mcg	0–100 mcg	100–200 mcg

*No DV has been established for these nutrients.

Appendix 9:

Body Mass Index Table

Height (inches) Weight (pounds)s

	BMI	58	59	60	61	62	63	64	65	66	67	68	69	70	71	72	73	74
Healthy Weight	19	91	94	97	100	104	107	110	114	118	121	125	128	132	136	140	144	148
	20	96	99	102	106	109	113	116	120	124	127	131	135	139	143	147	151	155
	21	100	104	107	111	115	118	122	126	130	134	138	142	146	150	154	159	163
	22	105	109	112	116	120	124	128	132	136	140	144	149	153	157	162	166	171
	23	110	114	118	122	126	130	134	138	142	146	151	155	160	165	169	174	179
	24	115	119	123	127	131	135	140	144	148	153	158	162	167	172	177	182	186
Overweight	25	119	124	128	132	136	141	145	150	155	159	164	169	174	179	184	189	194
	26	124	128	133	137	142	146	151	156	161	166	171	176	181	186	191	197	202
	27	129	133	138	143	147	152	157	162	167	172	177	182	188	193	199	204	210
	28	134	138	143	148	153	158	163	168	173	178	184	189	195	200	206	212	218
	29	138	143	148	153	158	163	169	174	179	185	190	196	202	206	213	219	225
	30	143	148	153	158	164	169	174	180	186	191	197	203	209	215	221	227	233
Obese	31	148	153	158	164	169	175	180	186	192	198	203	209	216	222	228	235	241
	32	153	158	163	169	175	180	186	192	198	204	210	216	222	229	235	242	249
	33	158	163	168	174	180	186	192	198	204	211	216	223	229	236	242	250	256
	34	162	168	174	180	186	191	197	204	210	217	223	230	236	243	250	257	264
	35	167	173	179	185	191	197	204	210	216	223	230	236	243	250	258	265	272
	36	172	178	184	190	196	203	209	216	223	230	236	243	250	257	265	272	280
	37	177	183	189	195	202	208	215	222	229	236	243	250	257	265	272	280	287
	38	181	188	194	201	207	214	221	228	235	242	249	257	264	272	279	288	295
	39	186	193	199	206	213	220	227	234	241	249	256	263	271	279	287	295	303
Very Obese	40	191	198	204	211	218	225	232	240	247	255	262	270	278	286	294	302	311
	41	196	203	209	217	224	231	238	246	253	261	269	277	285	293	302	310	319
	42	201	208	215	222	229	237	244	252	260	268	276	284	292	301	309	318	326
	43	205	212	220	227	235	242	250	258	266	274	282	291	299	308	316	325	334
	44	210	217	225	232	240	248	256	264	272	280	289	297	306	315	324	333	342
	45	215	222	230	238	246	254	262	270	278	287	295	304	313	322	331	340	350
	46	220	227	235	243	251	259	267	276	284	293	302	311	320	329	338	348	358
	47	224	232	240	248	256	265	273	282	291	299	308	318	327	338	346	355	365
	48	229	237	245	254	262	270	279	288	297	306	315	324	334	343	353	363	373
	49	234	242	250	259	267	278	285	294	303	312	322	331	341	351	361	371	381
	50	239	247	255	264	273	282	291	300	309	319	328	338	348	358	368	378	389
	51	244	252	261	269	278	287	296	306	315	325	335	345	355	365	375	386	396
	52	248	257	266	275	284	293	302	312	322	331	341	351	362	372	383	393	404
	53	253	262	271	280	289	299	308	318	326	338	348	358	369	379	390	401	412
	54	258	267	276	285	295	303	314	324	334	344	354	365	376	386	397	408	420

Appendix 9: Sample Menus in Approximate Calorie Ranges

1,600-Calorie Menu Gluten Free

Meals	Monday	Tuesday	Wednesday	Thursday	Friday	Saturday	Sunday
Breakfast	1 cup cooked rice or oat cereal w/tbsp. flax meal ¼cup walnuts ½cup blueberry Greek nonfat yogurt 1 cup strawberries Warm beverage	1 scoop Jay Robb's egg white protein powder 1 tbsp. flax meal 1 cup vanilla almond or soy milk 1 small banana ice/blend	1–2 Vann's toasted waffle 2 tbsp. peanut butter 1 tbsp. flax meal 1 tsp. jam 1 cup blueberries Warm beverage	1 hard- boiled egg cut into ½ sandwich on 1 piece of Udis whole grain bread toasted ¼sliced avocado 2 slices tomato ½ cup fresh OJ Warm beverage	1 cup cooked rice or millet cereal w/tbsp. flax ¼cup almonds ½ cup peach Greek nonfat yogurt ¼melon sliced Warm beverage	1 scoop protein powder 1 tbsp. flax meal 1 cup vanilla almond or soy milk 1 cup berries ice/blend	2 whole grain gluten-free pancakes (Cherrybrook Farms is a good brand) Topped w/cup of fresh fruit 1 scrambled egg Warm beverage
Lunch	3 oz. grilled chicken breast Small green salad w/lemon and oil 1 small red potato microwaved and cut into salad	Egg white omelet (4 egg whites) 1 oz. feta Sautéed spinach and mushrooms ½ large baked potato topped w/salsa	3 oz. turkey burger ½ large sweet potato Steamed asparagus w/lemon and drizzle oil	Leftover stir fry: 3 oz. lean beef w/veggies 1 cup cooked brown rice	Tacos: 3 oz. grilled chicken sliced into 2 rice or corn tortillas warmed ¼ sliced avocado Lettuce Salsa Tomatoes	3 oz. sliced turkey breast 2 slices toasted Udi's bread ¼ sliced avocado Tomato salad w/drizzle olive oil and oregano	3 oz. grilled salmon w/mustard and dill 1 cup cooked brown rice Steamed broccoli w/drizzle oil
Snack	½ cup nonfat peach Greek yogurt 1 small fruit	¼ cup raisins ¼ cup almonds 1 cup vanilla almond milk	½ cup nonfat blood orange Greek yogurt 1 small fruit	1 tbsp. peanut butter 1 apple	½ cup nonfat blueberry Greek yogurt 1 small fruit	½ cup nonfat peach Greek yogurt 1 small fruit	½ cup nonfat blood orange Greek yogurt 1 small fruit
Dinner	Spicy salmon / avocado or tuna roll Miso soup Seaweed salad	4 oz. turkey burger 1 cup cooked grain Steamed asparagus w/lemon and drizzle oil	Stir fry: 4 oz. lean beef Sautéed w/snow peas, carrots, broccoli, lemon, ginger, garlic, oil 1 cup cooked brown rice	Stir fry: 4 oz. lean beef Sautéed w/snow peas, carrots, broccoli, lemon, ginger, garlic, oil 1 cup cooked brown rice	4 oz. grilled salmon w/mustard and dill 1 cup lentil salad w/carrots and tomatoes Steamed asparagus w/lemon and drizzle oil	2 lamb chops (4 oz.) 1 cup mashed potatoes Steamed green beans w/drizzle oil	1 cup cooked gluten-free pasta topped w/4 oz. tuna Tbsp. pesto 1 tbsp. grated cheese Sautéed escarole w/garlic and oil

Appendix 9: Sample Menus in Approximate Calorie Ranges

1,600-Calorie Menu

Meals	Monday	Tuesday	Wednesday	Thursday	Friday	Saturday	Sunday
Breakfast	1 cup cooked oatmeal 1 cup nonfat Greek yogurt ½ cup berries Warm beverage	1 toaster waffle w/1 tsp. jam 2 hard-boiled egg whites 1 slice melon Warm beverage	½ cup low-fat cottage cheese 1 small whole-wheat pita toasted w/1 tsp. jam 1 slice melon Warm beverage	2 slices whole-grain toast 2 tbsps. peanut butter 1 tbsp. jam ½ cup fruit salad Warm beverage	1 cup whole-grain cereal 1 cup skim milk ¼ cup dried apricots Warm beverage	2 small buck-wheat pancakes topped w/ fresh fruit 1 cup nonfat Greek yogurt Warm beverage	1 cup cooked Kashi cereal 1 cup skim milk ¼ cup raisins Warm beverage
Am Snack	1 fruit 1 cup nonfat Greek yogurt	1 fruit 1 cup nonfat Greek yogurt	1 fruit 1 cup nonfat Greek yogurt	1 fruit ½ cup nonfat cottage cheese	1 fruit 1 cup nonfat Greek yogurt	If you sleep late on the weekend, you may not need a morning snack	
Lunch	Green salad w/ tomatoes, green beans other veggies 3 oz. can tuna ½ cup chickpeas 1 small whole-grain roll 1 tbsp. low-fat dressing	1 cup vegetable soup ½ turkey (3 oz.) sandwich on whole-grain bread Sliced avocado and tomato salad w/olive oil/ vinegar	Green salad w/pepper, tomatoes, etc. Vinaigrette 3 oz. poached salmon or grilled chicken 1 small red potato	Amy's vegetarian burrito (frozen) Small green salad w/low-fat dressing	Green salad w/tomatoes, green beans Vinaigrette 3 oz. can tuna ½ cup chickpeas 1 small red potato 1 tbsp. low-fat dressing	3 oz. grilled chicken wrapped in warm corn tortilla w/salsa and avocado 1 cup vegetable soup	1 cup turkey chili 1 slice melted cheese 1 cup cooked brown rice leftover veggies
Dinner	4 oz. lamb chop ½ cup couscous Sautéed escarole w/ garlic and olive oil	½ cup cooked brown rice 4 oz. poached salmon Steamed asparagus w/ drizzle olive oil and lemon	½cup cooked brown rice Stir-fried scallops (4 oz.), soy, ginger, garlic, lemon, broccoli, carrots, mushrooms	½ small microwaved sweet potato 4 oz. grilled chicken or fish Sautéed kale w/ garlic/olive oil	4 oz. steak ½ small baked potato Steamed broccoli and carrots w/bit of olive oil	1 cup turkey chili ½ cup cooked brown rice Sautéed spinach and mushrooms w/oil and garlic	Egg white omelet w/ mushroom Salad w/other veggies Oil/ vinegar 1 small red potato
Dessert	½ cup berries	Orange slices	½ cup pineapple chunks	½ cup fruit salad	1 slice melon	½ cup berries	½ cup fruit salad

Appendix 9: Sample Menus in Approximate Calorie Ranges

1,800-Calorie Menu

Meals	Monday	Tuesday	Wednesday	Thursday	Friday	Saturday	Sunday
Breakfast	1 cup cooked steel cut oats 1 cup nonfat apricot Greek yogurt ¼ cup walnuts ½ cup berries Warm beverage	1 small whole wheat pita toasted 1 hard boiled egg sliced into pita Sliced tomatoes 1 tbsp. pesto ½ cup fresh OJ Warm beverage	whole wheat toasted English muffin topped w/ 2 tbsp. peanut butter 1 tsp. jam ½ cup berries Warm beverage	1 cup cooked steel cut oats 1 cup nonfat apricot Greek yogurt ¼ cup walnuts ½ cup berries Warm beverage	½ cup low fat granola on top of fruited Greek yogurt ¼ cup walnuts ½ cup berries Warm beverage	Egg white omelet topped w/mushrooms 2 slices whole grain toast w/ jam 1 slice melon Warm beverage	Egg white omelet topped w/mushrooms 2 slices whole grain toast w/ jam 1 slice melon Warm beverage
Lunch	3–4 oz. turkey breast in small whole wheat pita Mustard side green 1 · salad w/tbsp. low-fat dressing	3 oz. can tuna over green salad w/lots of veggies ½ cup chickpeas 1 red potato microwaved and sliced into salad 1 tbsp. low-fat dressing	Egg white omelet topped w/veggies 1 red potato Sliced tomato and avocado salad w/bit of balsamic	3–4 oz. grilled chicken on bec of salad greens 1 small whole grain roll 1 tbsp. low-fat dressing	3–4 oz. lean roast beef ½ micro waved sweet potato Leftover broccoli	1 cup cooked leftover pasta 3–4 oz. shrimp Side salad of mixed greens w/tbsp. low-fat dressing	1 cup cooked leftover pasta 3–4 oz. shrimp Side salad of mixed greens w/tbsp. low-fat dressing
Afternoon Snack	1 small fruit 1 fruited Greek yogurt	1 small fruit ½ cup low fat cottage cheese	1 small fruit ½ cup low-fat cottage cheese	1 small fruit 1 oz. string cheese	1 small fruit 1 fruited Greek yogurt	1 small fruit ½ cup low-fat cottage cheese	1 small fruit ½ cup low-fat cottage cheese
Dinner	2 scrambled eggs 1–2 strips turkey bacon ½ baked potato w/pat butter Steamed brussels sprouts w/ drizzle olive oil	Chicken tacos: 4–5 oz. grilled chicken sliced into 3- 4 corn tortillas Shredded lettuce 1–2 oz. cheddar cheese Salsa Sliced avocado	4–5 oz. steak ½ baked potato w/pat butter Spinach salad w/low-fat dressing	4–5 oz. baked halibut ½ baked potato or sweet potato Steamed broccoli w/drizzle olive oil	1½ cups cooked pasta w/tomato sauce 4–5 oz. cooked shrimp Steamed asparagus w/drizzle olive oil	1½ cups turkey chili 1½ cups cooked brown rice Steamed green beans and carrots w/drizzle olive oil	1½ cups turkey chili 1½ cups cooked brown rice Steamed green beans and carrots w/drizzle olive oil
Dessert	1 cup berries	1 slice melon	1 cup berries	1 slice melon	Orange slices	1 cup berries	1 cup berries

Appendix 9: Sample Menus in Approximate Calorie Ranges

1,800-Calorie Menu-Lacto-Ovo Vegetarian

Meals	Monday	Tuesday	Wednesday	Thursday	Friday	Saturday	Sunday
Breakfast	Vann's toaster waffles 2 tbsp. peanut butter jam ½ cup berries Coffee	1 cup cooked instant oatmeal 1 cup nonfat Greek yogurt ¼ cup almonds 1 banana Coffee	1 cup Cheerios cereal 1 cup soy milk ¼ cup walnuts ½ cup berries Coffee	2 slices raisin bread toasted w/jam 2 tbsps. peanut butter jam 1 slice melon Coffee	1 cup instant oatmeal 1 cup nonfat Greek yogurt ¼ cup almonds 1 banana Coffee	Egg white omelet w/ veggies 1 toasted whole-grain English muffin w/jam 1 slice melon Coffee	2 small homemade Buckwheat pancakes (Arrowhead Mills) 1 tbsp. maple syrup or jam 1 scrambled egg ½ cup berries Coffee
Lunch	Big green salad w/ ½ cup chickpeas 1 slice swiss cheese Lots of other veggies 2 small red potatoes Light salad dressing w/balsamic and olive oil	1 slice cheese pizza w/extra veggies on top 1 cup vegetable soup	Spinach salad w/tomatoes, 1 hard boiled egg, ½ cup nonfat cottage cheese and light dressing 1 small whole grain roll	2 Morningstar Farms veggie burgers wrapped in whole wheat flour tortilla w/1 tbsp. hummus 1 bowl vegetable soup	Egg white omelet (1/2 cup Eggbeaters) w /Pam and sautéed zucchini/tomato	Amy's vegetarian burritos Bowl of vegetable soup	4 oz. stir- fried tofu 1 cup cooked brown rice Leftover veggies
Afternoon Snack	1 cup skim milk 1 fruit	1 cup nonfat Greek yogurt 1 slice melon	1 cup nonfat Greek yogurt 1 fruit	1 slice (1 oz.) cheese 1 apple	1 slice soy cheese	1 cup vanilla soy milk 1 fruit	1 cup nonfat Greek yogurt 1 fruit
Dinner	Egg white omelet w/ mushroom s 2 slices wholegrain toast w/jam Sautéed spinach w/garlic and oil	4 oz. stir fried tofu w/sesame seeds, garlic, oil, ginger, soy sauce, lemon, broccoli, carrots, snow peas 1½ cups cooked brown rice	1 cup cooked pasta w/tomato sauce 1 cup chickpeas Sautéed zucchini, mushrooms 2 tbsps. grated cheese	1½ cups vegetarian chili 1½ cups cooked brown rice Roasted asparagus and cauliflower w/ drizzle olive oil and onions	½ sweet potato Green salad w/light dressing 1 cup nonfat Greek yogurt 1 slice melon 4 oz. stir fried tofu w/sesame seeds, garlic, oil, ginger, soy sauce, lemon, broccoli, carrots, snow peas 1½ cups cooked brown rice	10 cheese ravioli w/tomato sauce Big green salad w/low-fat dressing 1 tbsp. grated cheese ½ cup fruit sorbet	2 bean and cheese burritos Sliced avocado and tomato salad
Dessert	1 cup berries	Slice melon	Orange slices	1 cup berries	Slice melon	Sliced mango	2 homemade cookies

**Appendix 9: Sample Menus in
Approximate Calorie Ranges**

2,100-Calorie (Pescetarian Vegetarian)

Meals	Monday	Tuesday	Wednesday	Thursday	Friday	Saturday	Sunday
Breakfast	2 whole-grain toaster waffles w/2 tbsps. maple syrup ½ cup low-fat cottage cheese ½ cup berries Sprinkle of pumpkin seeds Warm beverage	1 cup cooked oatmeal ¼ cup walnuts 1 cup nonfat vanilla Greek yogurt ½ banana Warm beverage	2 slices wholegrain toast 1 tbsp. jam ½cup scrambled eggbeaters w/ Pam 1 slice swiss cheese 1 slice melon Warm beverage	1 cup whole-grain cereal 1 cup vanilla almond milk ¼ cup almonds Handful raisins Warm beverage	1 whole-grain English muffin 2 tbsps. almond butter 1 cup skim milk Jam 1 slice melon Coffee	3 buckwheat waffles w/ maple syrup 1 scrambled organic egg Bowl of berries Warm beverage	Smoothie: 1 scoop Jay Robb vanilla protein powder 1 cup nonfat vanilla yogurt 1 banana Ice/ blend Small blueberry muffin
AM Snack	Granola bar 1 cup vanilla almond milk	1 fruit 1 wedge cheese	1 fruit 1 cup nonfat Greek yogurt w/nuts	1 granola bar 1 cup nonfat yogurt w/nuts	½ cup low-fat cottage cheese Sprinkle walnuts Fresh fruit	Handful trail mix 1 cup skim or vanilla almond milk	1 hard-boiled egg Whole grain crackers Hummus
Lunch	2 Garden burgers w/ cheese wrapped in 1 flour tortilla Tomato soup	Egg white omelet w/ veggies Small baked potato w/bit of butter Green salad whittle olive oil, balsamic, herbs	6 oz. marinated tofu on large whole-grain roll Big bowl minestrone soup	4 oz. Dr. Praeger's fish sticks 1½ cups cooked brown rice Steamed broccoli and carrots w/drizzle olive oil and lemon	1½ cups vegetarian chili w/1 slice melted cheese 1½ cups cooked brown rice Green salad w/ little olive oil, balsamic, herbs	4 oz. homemade tuna salad on large whole-grain roll w/ lettuce and tomato Big bowl soup	1 cup lentil soup w/1 slice melted cheese 1½ cups cooked brown rice Spinach salad w/tomatoes and avocado, dried cranberries and ¼ cup walnuts w/ dressing
Aft. Snack	1 fresh fruit 1 cup vanilla Greek yogurt granola	1 fresh fruit 1 cup almond milk handful trail mix	1 cup fruit salad ½ cup low-fat cottage cheese topped w/dried fruit and nuts	1 fresh fruit 1 cup vanilla Greek yogurt w/ sprinkle granola	1 fresh fruit 1 cup skim milk 1 packet oatmeal	1 banana 1 cup vanilla Greek yogurt Handful nuts	1 fresh fruit 1 wedge cheese crackers
Dinner	4–5 oz. Dr. Praeger's fish sticks 1½ cups mashed potatoes or baked potato or sweet potato fries sautéed spinach and mushrooms w/ garlic and oil	Grilled cheese (3 oz. cheese) sandwich w/ tomatoes Big bowl lentil or minestrone soup	2 cups cooked pasta w/4–5 oz. shrimp in tomato sauce Sautéed zucchini and carrots w/little olive-oil, lemon, herbs	1½ cups vegetarian chili w/melted cheese 1 ½ cups cooked brown rice Steamed broccoli and carrots w/drizzle olive oil	10 cheese ravioli w/tomato sauce Sautéed escarole w/ garlic, lemon, olive oil	Mexican: 3 bean burritos w/ beans and cheese 1½ cups cooked brown rice Green salad with low-fat dressing	Oriental stir-fry w/ 6 oz. tofu, lots of veggies 1½ cups cooked brown rice
Dessert	Fruit and yogurt topped w/nuts	Fruit and yogurt	1 cup fruit sorbet w/ cookies	Fruit and yogurt	Fresh fruit over frozen yogurt	Fruit and yogurt	1 cup frozen yogurt

Appendix 9: Sample Menus in Approximate Calorie Ranges

2,100-Calorie Menu

Meals	Monday	Tuesday	Wednesday	Thursday	Friday	Saturday	Sunday
Breakfast	1 cup cooked oatmeal 1 cup nonfat Greek yogurt ¼ cup walnuts ½ banana Warm beverage	2 slices wheat bread 2 tbsps. peanut butter 1 cup almond milk 1 slice melon Warm beverage	½ cup low-fat cottage cheese 1 slice melon 2 toaster waffles w/ bit of syrup Warm beverage	½ cup Grape Nuts cereal 1 cup vanilla almond milk ¼ cup almonds ½ banana Warm beverage	Smoothie made w/1 cup nonfat Greek yogurt, ½ banana 1 scoop protein powder Ice and blend	Egg white omelet w/ mushrooms 1 whole wheat roll toasted w/jam 1 slice melon Warm beverage	Breakfast Burrito: One warm whole wheat flour tortilla filled w/1 scrambled egg 1 oz. cheddar cheese Salsa ½ cup orange juice Warm beverage
Lunch	4 oz. grilled chicken breast wrapped in flour tortilla w/ lettuce, tomato, and avocado	4 oz. tuna salad on 2 slices whole wheat bread w/lettuce, tomato and avocado	4 oz. sliced turkey breast wrapped in whole wheat pita ¼ avocado sliced Sliced tomatoes Drizzle Italian dressing	Egg white omelet w/ veggies ½ large baked potato w/pat butter Salad w/bit of dressing	1½ cups cooked pasta salad w/4 oz. shrimp or chicken, tossed with cooked veggies Small green salad w/ dressing 1 tbsp. grated parmesan cheese	1 cup turkey or vegetarian chili 1 ½ cups cooked brown rice Green salad w/ olive oil based dressing	Bowl of lentil soup 2 slices cheddar cheese melted on toasted English muffin Small green salad w/bit of dressing
PM Snack (this could go in after lunch later in the afternoon or have the fresh fruit after dinner)	1 cup vanilla almond milk 1 small fruit	1 cup nonfat Greek yogurt 1 small fruit	1 oz. cheese 1 apple	Small handful raisins and nuts 1 cup vanilla almond milk	½ cup low-fat cottage cheese ½ cup berries	1 cup nonfat Greek yogurt ½ cup berries	½ cup low-fat cottage cheese ½ cup berries
Dinner	5 oz. beef stir fried w/broccoli/ mushrooms, snow peas, carrots Oil, lemon, tamari, sesame seeds, garlic 1 cup cooked brown rice	1½ cups turkey chili 1 cup cooked brown rice Roasted brussels sprouts w/garlic and oil	5 oz. poached salmon w/ mustard and dill 1 cup cooked brown rice Cooked greens w/ little olive oil, lemon, garlic	1 cup cooked pasta w/5 oz. shrimp sautéed w/garlic and oil, basil Steamed asparagus w/ lemon, herbs	5 oz. lean hamburger ½ sweet potato Steamed string beans and carrots w/olive oil and lemon	2 Garden Burgers ½ sweet potato Sautéed spinach w/ carrots/ garlic, oil, lemon	½ baked chicken breast (5 oz.) Sautéed zucchini, carrots, eggplant w/oil, lemon, herbs
Dessert	1 cup berries	1 slice melon	15 grapes	1 cup berries	Orange slices	½ cup frozen yogurt	½ cup fruit sorbet

Appendix 9: Sample Menus in Approximate Calorie Ranges

2,400-Calorie Menu

Meals	Monday	Tuesday	Wednesday	Thursday	Friday	Saturday	Sunday
Breakfast	2 slices whole grain bread 1 scrambled egg ½ cup berries Warm beverage	1 cup cooked oatmeal 1 cup nonfat Greek yogurt ½ cup OJ Warm beverage	1 cup whole grain cereal 1 cup skim milk 1 small fruit Warm beverage	½ cup low-fat cottage cheese topped w/ ¾ cup fruit salad Small blueberry muffin Warm beverage	2 toaster waffles w/syrup 1 scrambled egg ¾ cup fresh fruit salad Warm beverage	1 cup cooked oatmeal 1 cup yogurt ¾ cup fruit salad Warm beverage	½ cup low-fat granola 1 cup yogurt 1 banana Warm beverage
AM Snack	1 small fruit 1 oz. string cheese	1 small fruit 1 cup yogurt	1 small fruit 1 cup yogurt	1 small fruit 1 cup vanilla almond milk	1 small fruit 1 oz. string cheese	1 small fruit	1 small fruit
Lunch	4–6 oz. marinated and baked tofu over 1 cup cooked brown rice Lots of veggies	1 vegetarian burrito Small green salad w/low-fat dressing	1 bowl lentil soup Grilled cheese sandwich on whole grain bread Small green salad	2 vegetarian burgers wrapped in large whole wheat pita 1 slice swiss cheese Sliced avocado and tomato ½ cup nonfat cottage cheese	Sushi: 2 spicy tuna rolls 1 bowl miso soup Seaweed salad	4–6 oz. shrimp or other fish mixed with 1 cup cooked pasta salad Steamed broccoli w/ lemon and herbs	Egg white omelet (6 egg whites) w/veggies 2 slices whole grain toast w/jam Side green salad w/dressing
Aft. Snack	1 cup milk 1 small fruit	½ cup nonfat cottage cheese 1 small fruit	1 cup yogurt 1 small fruit	1 small fruit	1 slice swiss cheese 4–5 crackers ½ cup juice	1 cup yogurt 1 small fruit	½ cup nonfat cottage cheese 1 small fruit 5–6 crackers
Dinner	6 oz. grilled fish 1 baked potato w/nonfat sour cream Sautéed green beans w/garlic and oil	6 oz. sautéed shrimp w/garlic and oil over 1 ½ cups cooked linguini w/2 tbsps. grated cheese Sautéed broccoli rabe w/garlic and oil	2 vegetarian burgers ½ large sweet potato Steamed broccoli and cauliflower w/drizzle olive oil and lemon	6 oz. turkey burger w/one slice melted swiss on toasted whole wheat English muffin w/mustard/ketchup ½ sweet potato Steamed broccoli	Stir fry: 3 oz. tempeh sliced and sautéed w/snow peas, mushrooms, broccoli, carrots, ginger, garlic, lemon, olive oil, soy sauce 1½ cups cooked brown rice	12 cheese ravioli w/tomato sauce 2 tbsps. grated cheese Mesclun salad w/low-fat dressing	6 oz. grilled salmon 1½ cups cooked wild rice Steamed broccoli w/little bit of lemon/oil
Dessert	½ cup berries	1 slice melon	Orange slices	Sliced mango	1 cup berries	½ cup fruit sorbet	½ cup fruit sorbet

Appendix 9: Sample Menus in Approximate Calorie Ranges

2,400-Calorie Menu - Gluten Free

Meals	Monday	Tuesday	Wednesday	Thursday	Friday	Saturday	Sunday
Breakfast	½ cup low-fat wheat-free granola 1 cup low-fat Greek yogurt ¼ cup walnuts ½ banana Warm beverage	1 cup whole-grain wheat-free cereal 1 cup skim milk ¼ cup raisins ¼ cup almonds Warm beverage	2 slices whole-grain gluten-free toast 2 tbsps. peanut butter w/jam 1 small fruit Warm beverage	1 scrambled egg 1 whole-grain wheat-free English muffin w/touch of whipped butter ¾ cup fruit salad Warm beverage	1 whole-grain wheat-free bagel 1 oz. low-fat cream cheese 1 oz. smoked salmon ½ cup OJ Warm beverage	2 wheat-free toaster waffles w/syrup 1 scrambled egg ¾ cup fresh fruit salad Warm beverage	1 cup cooked oatmeal 1 cup low-fat Greek yogurt ¾ cup fruit salad Warm beverage
AM Snack	1 cup skim milk 1 fruit	1 cup low-fat Greek yogurt 1 fruit	½ cup low-fat cottage cheese 1 fruit	1 cup low-fat Greek yogurt 1 cup berries	1 oz. string cheese 1 fruit	1 apple 1–2 tbsps. Peanut butter	1/3 cup raisins and nuts
Lunch	1 small hamburger (4 oz.) on wheat-free roll w/mustard Green salad w/low-fat dressing	½ grilled chicken breast on bed of greens w/2 small red potatoes Low-fat dressing	4 oz. turkey breast on 2 slices gluten free bread w/mustard Sliced tomato and avocado salad w/balsamic vinegar	4 oz. tuna salad w/low-fat mayo On wheat-free roll Big bowl vegetable or minestrone soup	Big salad w/4 oz. shrimp 1 ½ cups cooked brown rice Low-fat dressing	4 oz. roast beef on gluten free bread (2 slices) w/mustard Green salad w/low-fat dressing	4 oz. poached salmon on bed of sautéed greens 1½ cups cooked brown rice Steamed asparagus or broccoli
Afternoon Snack	1 cup milk ½ cup whole-grain cereal 1 small fruit	1 oz. string cheese 1 small fruit 3–4 wheat-free crackers	1 cup yogurt 1 small fruit ½ cup whole-grain gluten-free cereal	1 glass soy milk 1 small fruit 1 toaster wheat waffle	1 slice swiss cheese 4–5 crackers ½ cup juice	1 cup yogurt 1 small fruit ½ cup low-fat wheat-free granola	½ cup nonfat cottage cheese one small fruit 3–4 wheat free crackers
Dinner	5 oz. grilled fish 1 baked potato w/nonfat sour cream Sautéed green beans w/garlic and oil	5 oz. sautéed shrimp w/garlic and oil over 1 cup gluten free linguini w/2 tbsps. grated cheese Sautéed broccoli rabe w/garlic and oil	5 oz. filet mignon or roast beef 1 baked sweet potato Sautéed spinach w/garlic and oil	5 oz. turkey burger w/one slice melted swiss on toasted wheat-free English muffin w/mustard/ketchup ½ sweet potato Steamed broccoli	½ grilled chicken breast (5 oz.) Sautéed escarole w/garlic and oil ¾ cup rice	10 cheese gluten-free Ravioli w/tomato sauce 2 tbsps. grated cheese Mesclun salad w/low-fat dressing	4–5 oz. tuna salad w/low-fat mayo on 2 slices wheat-free bread 1 cup vegetable soup
Dessert	1 cup berries	1 slice melon	Orange slices	Sliced mango	1 cup berries	2 homemade cookies	½ cup frozen yogurt

Appendix 9: Sample Menus in Approximate Calorie Ranges

2,700-Calorie Menu

Meals	Monday	Tuesday	Wednesday	Thursday	Friday	Saturday	Sunday
Breakfast	2 whole-grain frozen toaster waffles 2 tbsps. Peanut butter 1 tbsp. jam 1 cup rice dream or almond milk 1 slice melon Warm beverage	1½ cups cooked oatmeal 1 cup nonfat Greek yogurt ¼ cup walnuts or almonds 1 cup berries Warm beverage	1 large whole wheat pita stuffed w/ scrambled egg whites (4) and spinach 1 cup chopped fruit Warm beverage	2 scrambled organic eggs cooked w/Pam spray and added veggies 2 slices spelt toast w/jam 1 slice melon Warm beverage	1½ cups whole-grain cereal 1 cup nonfat Greek yogurt ¼ cup walnuts 1 banana Warm beverage	3 whole wheat pancakes ¼ cup syrup ½ cup berries 1 scrambled organic egg Warm beverage	3 slices french toast w/ ¼ cup syrup 4 scrambled egg whites 1 cup berries Warm beverage
AM Snack	1 fruit ½ cup low-fat cottage cheese	1 fruit l cup nonfat Greek yogurt	1 fruit 1 cup rice dream	1 fruit 1 cup nonfat Greek yogurt	1 fruit ½ cup low-fat cottage cheese	1 fruit ¼ cup almonds	1 fruit 1cup nonfat Greek yogurt
Lunch	6 oz. grilled chicken breast over romaine greens w/other veggies 2 small microwaved red potatoes Balsamic dressing	6 oz. chicken salad made with canola oil mayo and mustard on 2 slices whole spelt bread Bowl of vegetable soup	Big beef and bean burrito with wheat flour tortilla Salsa Sliced tomatoes and ¼ sliced avocado w/ balsamic dressing	6 oz. roast beef on rye w/ mustard Green salad w/olive oil-based dressing	6 oz. grilled chicken breast wrapped in large whole wheat flour tortilla Green salad w/ olive oil based dressing	6 oz. lean burger on whole-grain roll Ketchup/ mustard Steamed broccoli w/ lemon/herbs	1 ½ cups vegetarian chili 1 oz. shredded cheddar 2 cups cooked brown rice Sautéed greens w/lemon and oil
Afternoon Snack	1 scoop protein powder (14 grams protein) 1 cup vanilla almond milk 1 banana	1 fruit 1 cereal bar 1 cup vanilla almond milk	1 scoop protein powder 1 cup vanilla almond milk 1 banana	1 fruit 1 cup nonfat Greek yogurt ¼ cup grape nuts cereal	1 scoop protein powder 1 cup rice dream 1 banana	1 fruit 1 oz. whole wheat pretzels 1 oz. string cheese	1 scoop protein powder 1 cup vanilla almond milk 1 banana
Dinner	1 big baked sweet potato topped w/pat butter 6 oz. grilled fish Sautéed broccoli rabe in oil and garlic	2 cups cooked brown rice 6 oz. spicy scallops w/soy and ginger Sautéed broccoli, carrots, mushrooms, water chestnuts	2 cups cooked rigatoni 6 oz. grilled chicken breast Black olives, capers, olive oil, garlic, sundried tomatoes Green salad	1 big baked potato topped w/pat butter 6–3 oz. turkey burger Steamed asparagus w/ lemon and oil Sliced tomatoes	12 cheese ravioli Tomato sauce 2 tbsp. parmesan cheese Sautéed zucchini, eggplant, mushrooms	2 cups vegetarian chili 1 oz. shredded cheddar 2 cups cooked brown rice Salad w/olive oil based dressing	6 oz. sautéed scallops 2 cups cooked risotto or plain rice Sautéed spinach and mushrooms
Dessert	1½ cups berries	2 slices melon	Orange slices	Sliced mango and strawberries	1½ cups berries	1 slice chocolate cake	1 cup frozen yogurt

Appendix 9: Sample Menus in Approximate Calorie Ranges

2,700-Calorie Menu

Meals	Monday	Tuesday	Wednesday	Thursday	Friday	Saturday	Sunday
Breakfast	2 whole-grain frozen waffles ¼cup maple syrup 1 scrambled egg 1 slice melon Warm beverage	2 slices whole-grain toast w/ 2 tbsps. peanut butter Jam 1 cup nonfat yogurt 1 banana Warm beverage	1 whole wheat pita stuffed w/ scrambled egg whites and 1 slice low-fat swiss ½ cup chopped fruit Warm beverage	1 cup cooked oatmeal w/1/4 cup Grape nuts 1 cup vanilla soy milk ¼ cup almonds ¼ cup raisins Warm beverage	2–3 oz. cereal 1 cup skim milk ¼cup walnuts 1 banana Warm beverage	3 whole wheat pancakes ¼ cup syrup ½cup berries 1 scrambled egg Warm beverage	3 slices french toast with ¼ cup maple syrup 1 cup nonfat yogurt w/ ½ cup berries Warm beverage
AM Snack	1 fruit 1 cup yogurt	1 fruit 1 cup soy milk	1 fruit 1 cup yogurt	1 fruit 1 cup yogurt	1 fruit 1 cup yogurt	1 fruit ¼cup almonds	1 fruit 1 cup soy milk
Lunch	1 turkey burger (5–6 oz.) 1 English muffin Green salad w/ olive oil- based dressing	5–6 oz. poached salmon 1 cup cooked risotto Steamed asparagus w/ lemon and bit of oil	2 Amy's California burgers wrapped in whole wheat flour tortilla ¼ avocado Salsa Sliced tomatoes	5–6 oz. roast beef on rye w/ mustard Green salad w/olive oil based dressing	5–6 oz. grilled chicken breast wrapped in whole wheat flour tortilla Green salad w/ olive oil based dressing	5–6 oz. tuna salad made with canola oil mayo and mustard on 2 slices whole-wheat bread Big bowl of vegetable soup	1½ cups turkey chili 1 cup cooked brown rice Sautéed greens w/lemon and oil
Afternoon Snack	1 fruit 1 cup yogurt 1 cereal bar	1 fruit 1 cereal bar 1 cup yogurt	1 fruit 1 cup milk ½cup low-fat granola	1 fruit ½ cup cottage cheese ½ cup low-fat granola	1 apple 1 slice cheese 4–5 whole wheat crackers	1 fruit 1 oz. pretzels 1 cup milk	1 fruit 1 cup yogurt ½ cup cereal
Dinner	1 large baked sweet potato 6 oz. grilled chicken breast Sautéed broccoli rabe in oil and garlic	1½ cups cooked brown rice 6 oz. spicy scallops w/soy and ginger Sautéed broccoli, carrots, mushrooms, water chestnuts	1½ cups cooked rigatoni 6 oz. chicken breast Black olives, capers, olive oil, garlic, sundried tomatoes Green salad	1 large baked potato 6 oz. filet mignon Steamed asparagus w/ lemon and oil Sliced tomatoes	12 cheese ravioli Tomato sauce 2 tbsp. parmesan cheese Sautéed zucchini, eggplant, mushrooms	1½ cups turkey chili 1½ cups cooked brown rice Salad w/olive oil based dressing	6 oz. sautéed shrimp 1½ cups cooked rice Sautéed spinach and mushrooms
Dessert	1½ cups berries	2 slices melon	Orange slices	Sliced mango and strawberries	1½ cups berries	1 chocolate brownie	1 cup frozen yogurt

Appendix 9: Sample Menus in Approximate Calorie Ranges

3,000-Calorie Menu

Meals	Monday	Tuesday	Wednesday	Thursday	Friday	Saturday	Sunday
Breakfast	1 whole-grain muffin 1 cup yogurt 1 piece of fruit Warm beverage	1½ cup oatmeal 1 cup yogurt ¼ cup nuts 1 banana Warm beverage	1 whole-grain muffin 1 cup yogurt 1 piece of fruit Warm beverage	2 slices whole-grain bread 2 tbsps. peanut butter w/jam ½ banana 1 cup milk Warm beverage	2–3 oz. cereal 1 cup skim milk ½ banana ¼ cup almonds Warm beverage	1½ cup oatmeal 1 cup yogurt ¼ cup nuts ½ cup stewed apricots and prunes Warm beverage	1 small bialy 1–2 oz. low-fat cream cheese Sliced smoked salmon 1 slice melon Warm beverage
AM Snack	1 fruit 1 cup yogurt	1 fruit 1 cup yogurt	1 fruit 1 cup yogurt	1 fruit 1 cup yogurt	1 fruit 1 cup yogurt	1 fruit 1 cup yogurt	1 fruit 1 cup yogurt
Lunch	4–5 oz. turkey wrap w/roasted red peppers Big salad w/ olive oil/vinegar/ mustard 1 cup vegetable soup	3 oz. plain tuna in big salad w/ lots of veggies ½ c. sliced tofu or beans 2 sm. red potatoes Olive oil/vinegar/ mustard dressing 1 cup lentil soup	Grilled turkey burger or regular burger (4–5 oz.) 1 whole wheat roll Mustard Big salad w/lots of veggies Olive oil/vinegar/ mustard dressing 1 cup minestrone soup	½ grilled chicken breast (4–5 oz.) 1 cup pasta salad Big salad w/lots of veggies Olive oil/vinegar/ mustard dressing 1 cup Minestrone soup	Egg white omelet w/2 slices cheese cooked w/oil Steamed veggies w/lemon, soy, mustard 1 whole wheat roll 1 bowl split pea soup	4–5 oz. Stir-fried shrimp with olive oil, garlic, tamari, lemon, broccoli, carrots, mushrooms 1 cup brown rice	2 cups mild vegetarian chili w/2 slices melted cheese Nonfat sour cream 1 cup brown rice Big salad w/lots of veggies Olive oil/vinegar/ mustard dressing
Afternoon Snack	1 cereal bar ½ cup cottage cheese 1 fruit	½ cup cottage cheese 5 whole grain crackers 1 fruit	1 cup yogurt 1 oz. cereal 1 fruit	1 cereal bar 1 cup yogurt 1 fruit	3 tbsps. hummus 5–6 whole grain crackers 1 slice cheese ½ cup juice	½ cup cottage cheese 5 whole grain crackers 1 fruit	1 cup yogurt 1 oz. cereal ½ banana
Dinner	8 oz. grilled fish 1½ cups brown rice Sautéed spinach Salad w/low-fat dressing	8 oz. grilled chicken 1½ cups cooked pasta w/olive oil and garlic 1 tbsp. grated cheese Steamed broccoli and carrots w/oil and lemon	2 shrimps fajitas Little guacamole 1 tbsp. sour cream Salad w/low-fat dressing	8 oz. spicy scallops 1½ cups brown rice Steamed mixed veggies	15 cheese ravioli Olive oil and garlic or pesto 1 tbsp. grated cheese Sautéed escarole w/garlic and oil	8 oz. turkey burger on Whole wheat English muffin Steamed broccoli and carrots w/oil and lemon	8 oz. filet mignon 1 large sweet potato Green beans w/lemon and oil
Dessert	Sliced apple	2 cups berries	3 slices melon	Orange slices	Sliced apple	1 slice chocolate cake	1½ cups frozen yogurt

**Appendix 10: Power Food Combos for Dancers
(Protein, Carbohydrate, and Fat)**

Breakfast Combos:
Scrambled eggs or whites w/toast and fresh fruit Oatmeal w/Greek yogurt and
fresh fruit
Whole-grain cereal w/vanilla almond milk, berries, and sliced almonds
Whole-grain English muffin topped w/peanut butter and jam and a glass of skim
milk Low-fat cottage cheese w/fresh fruit and whole-grain toast

Lunch Options:
Tuna salad sandwich on whole wheat bread topped w/avocado and tomato
Green salad topped w/grilled chicken or salmon w/dressing and whole-grain roll
Peanut butter and jelly sandwich, glass of milk, banana
Bean and cheese burrito w/side salad
Veggie burger topped w/one slice swiss cheese on whole-grain bun topped w/
lettuce and tomato

Dinner Combos:
Turkey chili over brown rice and steamed broccoli Grilled chicken or fish over cous-
cous w/sautéed kale
Turkey meatballs and spaghetti w/tomato sauce and big green salad
Sliced steak w/baked potato and sautéed spinach and mushrooms
Egg white omelet w/veggies, microwaved sweet potato and steamed asparagus
Marinated tofu baked and served with brown rice and sautéed collard greens

Snacks for Energy:
Hard-boiled egg and baby carrots Handful raisins and nuts
Greek yogurt and fruit String cheese and apple
Luna and Kind Bars are okay - drink with plenty of water

Bibliography

American Dietetic Association. www.eatright.org.

American College of Sports Medicine, Exercise Guidelines. www.acsm.org.

Changes to the Nutrition Facts label. www.fda.gov/Food/GuidanceRegulation/GuidanceDocumentsRegulatoryInformation.

Colbin, Annemarie. Food and Healing. Ballantine Books, 1996.

Coleman, Ellen. Cardiovascular Nutrition and Fitness. Nutrition Dimension, Inc., 2004.

Coleman, Ellen. Diet, Exercise and Fitness. Nutrition Dimension, Inc., 2002.

Guidance or Industry: A Food Labeling Guide (14. Appendix F: Calculate the percent Daily Value for the Appropriate Nutrients), January 2013. www.fda.gov/Food/GuidanceRegulation/GuidanceDocumentsRegulatoryInformation.

Gustafson, Nancy. Osteoporosis Prevention & Treatment. Nutrition Dimension, Inc., 2010.

Katch, Frank & McArdle, William. Nutrition. Weight Control and Exercise. Lea & Febiger, 7th Edition, 2010.

Kay, Leslie. Alternative and Complementary Nutrition Therapy. Nutrition Dimension, Inc., 2005.

Kobriger, Annette M. How The Brain Affects Food Intake. Nutrition Dimension, Inc., 2006.

Kupper, Cynthia. Gluten Intolerance and GI Disorders. Nutrition Dimension, Inc., 2008.

Linder, Maria. Nutritional Biochemistry and Metabolism with Clinical Applications. Elsevier, 1991.

USDA. www.choosemyplate.gov/2015-2020-dietary-guidelines-answers-your-questions.

We Can! Ways to Enhance Children's Activity & Nutrition. www.wecan.nhlbi.nih.gov.

Whitney, Eleanor, & Rolfes, Sharon. Understanding Nutrition. 14th Edition, 2016.

ACKNOWLEDGEMENTS

I would like to acknowledge my husband, Rick, and my family whose love and support I could not do without, as well as the inspiration I have received from my mentors and teachers along my path, including Luigi, Jean Paul Mustone, Frank Pietri, and Lianne Plane.

Photograph Credits:

Cover- Master 1305 Studios

Interior- The photographers whose work is represented on Shutterstock, RawPixel, Unsplashed, Pexels, Allison Marras, Jodie Morgan, Mariana Medvedeva, Michael Mroczek, Mitchell Hollander, Nino Liverani, Naya Stoica, Ola Mishchenko, Sudeera Senevirante, Taylor Kiser, Victor Freitas, Julenocheck, Korrapon Karapan, Wisa Thananimit, Una Shimpraga, Africa Studio, Master 1305 Studios, Mas Anyanka, Focal Point, Crevis Photo, LightField Studios, Jinning Li, Alex Skopje, StudioPhotoD Florez, Baibaz, Kucher AV, Mara Ze, Olena Yakobchuk